NEUROGENIC
COMMUNICATION
DISORDERS

NEUROGENIC COMMUNICATION DISORDERS

Aphasia and Cognitive-Communication Disorders

By

SAKINA S. DRUMMOND, Ph.D.

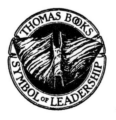

CHARLES C THOMAS • PUBLISHER, LTD.
Springfield • Illinois • U.S.A.

Published and Distributed Throughout the World by

CHARLES C THOMAS • PUBLISHER, LTD.
2600 South First Street
Springfield, Illinois 62704

ISBN 0-398-07650-2 (hard)
ISBN 0-398-07651-0 (paper)

Library of Congress Catalog Card Number: 2006040450

With THOMAS BOOKS *careful attention is given to all details of manufacturing and design. It is the Publisher's desire to present books that are satisfactory as to their physical qualities and artistic possibilities and appropriate for their particular use.* THOMAS BOOKS *will be true to those laws of quality that assure a good name and good will.*

Printed in the United States of America
MM-R-3

Library of Congress Cataloging-in-Publication Data

Drummond, Sakina S.
  Neurogenic communication disorders : aphasia and cognitive-communication disorders
/ by Sakina S. Drummond.
     p. ; cm.
  Includes bibliographical references and index.
  ISBN 0-398-07650-2 (hard) -- ISBN 0-398-07651-0 (pbk.)
     1. Communicative disorders. 2. Aphasia. 3. Cognition disorders. I. Title.
  [DNLM: 1. Communication Disorders. 2. Aphasia. WL 340.2 D795n 2006]
  RC423.D78 2006
  362.196'855--dc22   2006040450

To: Buggle–Emo–Raja–Tiny

PREFACE

This text is the culmination of my insatiable curiosity to understand the relationship between brain functions and communication, and years of teaching-learning and clinical experiences. Although the brain has been acknowledged as a fascinating organ, it represents the essence of who and what we are as a species. The brain regulates all bodily functions and behaviors—one of which is communication. An understanding of human communication requires working knowledge of basic neuroscience, which involves the study of normal neural structures and mechanisms at both macroscopic and microscopic levels. This knowledge serves as the foundation for the diagnosis and management of anomalous functions in the clinical fields of neurology and speech-language pathology. Clinical preparation in each of these professions requires a comprehensive appreciation of the brain-behavior connection and consequences of brain dysfunction on human communication.

The text begins with a review of core concepts relating to the structures and interrelated functions of the brain; this information serves as the precursor to understanding the possible causes and nature of neurogenic communication disorders and related clinical issues. It also includes options for assessing the prevailing communication disorder and highlights the association between the etiologies and underlying neuropathology to overt communication symptoms; the rationale for their presentation is to foster essential critical thinking skills to derive at differential diagnosis and formulate a prognosis for recovery of the identified symptoms. The text ends with the offering of diverse management and treatment options that strive to either restore or stabilize the impaired communication and related functions.

The presented information has selectively focused on the description of language and cognitive-communication disorders secondary to brain lesions. The text aims to guide students and professionals who diagnose, explain, and implement rehabilitation strategies for individuals with acquired neurogenic communication disorders. This objective is reflected in its elaboration of disrupted decoding and encoding of linguistic units such as symbols (words) representing semantics and morphology (meaningful units), and the rules (syntax and pragmatics) for using them during communication. The interconnectivity between language and cognition is stressed through establishing the influence of perceptual and cognitive functions on language/communication modalities of comprehension and production. Contributions from the fields of neuro- and psycholinguistics have been incorporated to help characterize and distinguish disorders such as aphasia, dementia, as well as traumatic brain injury and nondominant (right) hemisphere lesions. The text shares insights some of which are contrary to conventional ideologies; it has also made a discernable effort to refrain from entering into any provocative discussion on issues regarding the nature of human "mind" (psyche) or any psychiatric disorders.

The content presentation has considered contemporary reading and learning preferences as well. Every attempt has been made to provide pertinent information in a simplified format with key concepts being italicized in their preliminary contextual descriptions. Diagrams and tables are utilized for the visual learner with balanced attention to the need for specificity and comprehensiveness with simultaneous tempering of redundant information. I remain sensitive to the perennial perception that neuroscience and related communication disorders is a nemesis to students in the field of communication disorders; it is my sincere hope that not only will this text help alleviate any apprehensiveness toward this exciting and challenging topic, but that it will serve as an initiation to the quest for knowledge and undaunting curiosity.

Sakina S. Drummond, Ph.D.

CONTENTS

ILLUSTRATIONS

Tables

NEUROGENIC
COMMUNICATION
DISORDERS

Chapter 1

DEVELOPMENT AND DESCRIPTION OF THE BRAIN

The human nervous system is organized into two components: a *central* (CNS) and *peripheral* (PNS) nervous system. This chapter focuses on the CNS, which includes the *brain* and the *spinal cord* each of which are encased by two different sets of protective tissues. The outer encasing is composed of a bony framework; the chain of bones, or the *vertebral column,* and protects the spinal cord while the brain is housed within the *cranium* (or skull). The inner protective casing is composed of three *meninges,* or layers of connective tissues (see Figure 5.2), which are organized in the following order:

- The *duramater,* implying "tough mother," is the outermost layer which is almost leathery in texture. It is further divided into an outer, *periosteal layer,* and the inner, *meningeal layer.* The gap between the duramater and the bony cranium is called the *epidural space.*
- The middle layer, the *arachnoid mater* appears "spider/web-like" because this translucent layer is infested by crisscrossing blood vessels. The space between the arachnoid and duramater is identified as the *subdural space,* however, the Anatomical Terminology Conference in 1997 has determined that this space is not readily identified except in the presence of a *hematoma* (or blood clot).
- The innermost *pia mater,* or "soft mother," is a fragile thin layer encasing the neural tissue. The space between the pia and arachnoid mater is termed the *subarachnoid space;* it is filled with the colorless *cerebrospinal fluid* (CSF).

The remainder of this chapter provides a review of the development of the different levels and structures that collectively form the human brain. It also describes the functions ascribed to these structures in a fully developed (adult) brain with the intent that such information will provide an appreciation of the complexity of the neural circuitry and processes, as well as its potential for disrupting human communication behaviors in the presence of some disease or pathology.

BRAIN DEVELOPMENT

The development of the human brain has its foundation in the concepts of phylogeny and ontogeny. *Phylogeny* relates to the genetic evolution or developmental patterns between species. *Ontogeny* describes the development of the fertilized ovum from a unicellular to multicellular organism within a given species. The ontogenic development of the human brain as it progresses from *embryonic* (first 8 weeks of gestation) to *fetal* (after 9 weeks) changes are depicted in Figures 1.1 and 1.2, and they have been described through the following stages (Table 1.1):

1st week: The fertilized, single cellular ovum (or *zygote*) undergoes *mitosis* (cell division) at the rate of 50,000 cells per minute. The embryo appears as a hollow ball, or *blastocyst,* consisting of an outer cell mass that later forms the placenta, and an inner cell mass that evolves into a fetus in the later stages. Within two hours after fertilization, the embryo begins to distinguish the left from right side. Around day three, eight undifferentiated cells capable of becoming any structure are identified. Before the end of the first week about 100–150 of these undifferentiated cells are commonly described as embryonic stem cells.

3rd week: At this stage, the embryo is called the *gastrula* and it displays a distinctive organization of its cells as three *germinal* layers. The descendants of these germinal layers will ultimately form different tissues and organs of the human body. The internal germinal layer, *endoderm,* will develop into the visceral organs including the pancreas, bladder, urethria, thyroid, lungs, and the liver. The middle, *mesodermal layer* will form the muscle (smooth, striated and cardiac), connective tissues (including the bone), and the vascular system (heart and blood vessels). The cells in the outer, *ectodermal layer* will develop into the nervous system, skin, including hair and nails, as well as the eyes and ears. During the third week, some ectodermal cells segregate to form

1 ¹/₂ mm long *neural plate,* which is the first sign of an evolving nervous system. The medial indented portion is identified as the *neural groove* and the raised edges as *neural folds.* The neural plate continues to develop so that the neural folds rise to form two lateral *neural ridges* almost encircling a medial *neural groove.* Two clusters of cells at the neck of the neural groove are identified as *neural crest.*

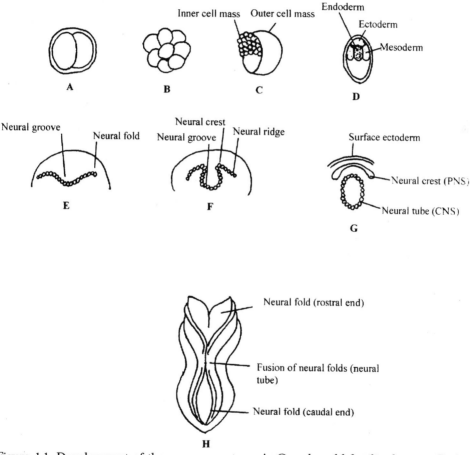

Figure 1.1. Development of the nervous system. A. One-day old fertilized ovum. B. At three days. C. Blastocyst at 5–6 days (transverse section). D. Gastrula with the three germinal layers (2–3 weeks). E. Formation of neural plate and two prominent landmarks (transverse section). F. Development of neural ridges and neural crests (transverse section). G. Mid-line fusion of neural folds resulting in formation of neural tube and separation of neural crest (transverse section). H. Dorsal view of the embryo at 4 weeks depicting the unfused rostral and caudal ends of the neural folds along with its central portion.

4th week: The cells of neural ridges continue to multiply and merge with the medial ward to form a *neural tube.* This stage is the first indication of a CNS that will ultimately develop in a brain and spinal cord. There is evidence to indicate that pregnant women exposed to heat, hot tubs, fever, saunas, etc. during the first eight weeks are more likely to deliver a baby with neural tube defect (e.g., Spina Bifida). The cells of the neural crest are left outside the neural tube to later evolve into the PNS to represent the cranial and spinal nerves and their sensory ganglia, as well as the efferent components of the *Autonomic Nervous System.*

Several structural developments occur around this period. First, the neural tube enlarges to form three regions:

- Its large rostral, or *cephalic* end landmarks the development of the brain. This end continues to grow to form the three primary subdivisions of the brain: the *rhombencephalon,* or the "hindbrain;" the *mesencephalon,* or the "midbrain;" and the *prosencephalon,* or the "forebrain."
- The narrow *caudal,* or tail end will elongate to form the spinal cord.
- The lumen, or inner *neural canal,* will become the *ventricles* in the brain and *central canal* of the spinal cord.

Around this period the cells in the neural tube also organize themselves in three layers (zones):

- The internal *ependymal* layer, which will later form the internal lining of the neural tube and the *choroid plexus.*
- The intermediate *mantle* layer forms the *gray matter* to later specialize as the *neurons* and *neuroglia.*
- The external *marginal* layer forms the *white matter* that will ultimately form the *nerve fibers* and *tracts.*

The cells in the anterior (ventral) region of neural tube, or the *basal lamina,* will later give rise to the motor and efferent pathways of pons, medulla and the cerebral peduncles. Correspondingly, the cells in the posterior (dorsal) region of the neural tube, or *alar lamina,* will give rise to the sensory and afferent components of the cranial nerves, as well as the cerebellum and its peduncles, and structures of the diencephalon and the telencephalon.

5–6 weeks: The cells within the rhombencephalon and the prosencephalon proliferate and each of these structures further organize into two distinct subdivisions. The rhombencephalon divides into the *mye-*

lencephalon, termed the *medulla oblongata* at birth, and the *metencephalon,* which will later differentiate into the pons and the cerebellum. The prosencephalon also subdivides into the *diencephalon* (the "intermediate brain") to give rise to the optic vesicles, and the *telencephalon* (the "endbrain"), which marks the origin of the cerebral hemispheres. Each of these developments also require the neural canal to undergo alterations which are later reflected in the formation of the ventricles of the brain.

10–12 weeks (2 ½ months): The 6th through 12th week of gestation is perhaps the most active period for the development of the nervous system. During this latter part of first trimester, the undifferentiated *stem cells* are the most versatile, and they rapidly organize themselves to form specific structures at different levels of the brain. For example, the metencephalon is now subdivided into the *pons* and the *cerebellum.* This stage marks the development of the *brainstem,* which clinically includes the medulla, pons, midbrain, and the emerging signs of cranial nerves at each of these levels as well. These structures however, are microscopic since the entire fetus is merely three inches long.

The cells within the diencephalon continue to subdivide to form several structures:

- The *thalamus* arises from the thickening of the alar plate on each side.
- The *epithalamus,* which will later form the pineal body and the posterior commissure.
- The *metathalamus* will differentiate into the medial and lateral geniculate bodies.
- The *hypothalamus* emerges from the lower part of the alar plate, and it will later include the mammillary bodies, the infundibulum, and the hypo/neurophysis (pituitary body).
- The *subthalamus* will evolve as the subthalamic nucleus.

During this period, the telencephalon also subdivides into the *rhinencephalon, corpus striatum,* and the *cerebral cortex.*

24 weeks (6 months): The cerebral cortex has evolved to form the two *cerebral hemispheres,* and they begin to show the presence of sulci and gyri. Rudimentary structures for hearing and vision begin to emerge, and there are signs of myelination of the white matter.

7–9 months (3rd trimester): There is a rapid development and refinement of the prosencephalon; this is reflected through the brain's hunger for consuming as much fats as possible. Although it is difficult to pinpoint a specific timetable for the formation of different structures, some of the obvious highlights of this stage include:

- Enlargement of the cerebral cortex.
- Demarcation of the *cerebral lobes* in each hemisphere.
- Development of the *anterior* and *posterior commissures* and the *corpus callosum,* each of which interconnect the right and left hemispheres.

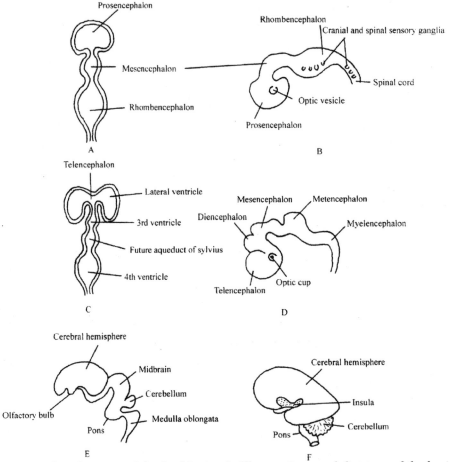

Figure 1.2. Development of the fetal brain. A. Three primary subdivisions of the brain. B. Lateral view of the brain at 4 weeks. C. Organization of the ventricles during the first trimester. D. Lateral view depicting subdivisions of the prosencephalon (telencephalon) and the rhombencephalon (metencephalon and myelencephalon). E. The brain at six months. F. The brain during the third trimester.

Table 1.1. Milestones Reflecting the Development of the Brain.

Age	Structures
3rd day	Eight undifferentiated cells
1st week	Blastocyst (inner and outer cell mass)
3rd week	Gastrula: three germinal layers (endoderm, mesoderm & ectoderm)
18th day	Neural plate → neural folds (and ridges) and neural groove
25th day	Neural tube (CNS) and neural crest (PNS)
4 weeks	Neural tube → brain + spinal cord + ventricles; 3 cellular layers (ependymal, mantle & marginal); basal and alar laminae Brain (rhombencephalon, mesencephalon and prosencephalon
5–6 weeks	Rhombencephalon → myelencephalon + metencephalon Prosencephalon → diencephalon + telencephalon
10–12 weeks	Metencephalon → pons and cerebellum Presence of primitive "brainstem" Formation of all cranial nerves, except I and II Evidence of 4 ventricles and central canal Diencephalon → thalamus, hypothalamus, epi-, meta-, and subthalamus Telencephalon → rhinencephalon, corpus striatum and cerebral cortex
24 weeks (6 months)	Presence of cerebral hemispheres
7–9 months	Demarcation of 5 cerebral lobes Commissures (anterior & posterior) + corpus callosum
At Birth	All structures developed; brain weight = 350 gm
At 20 years	Brain weight = 1400 gm

At Birth: The brain weighs 350 gm, but it triples in size in the first year of life. The increase in weight results are due to several factors:
- Establishment and myelination of tracts
- Formation of new synaptic connections
- Proliferation of glial cells in the gray matter.

A recent report on the study of brain circumference of children with autism indicates that these children have smaller head circumference at birth, but they show a sudden and excessive increase in head size during the first year. The rapid growth was primarily observed in the frontal cortex, and was speculated to generate excessive "neural noise," which the infant was unable to cope with, and thus attributed to the observed withdrawal behaviors among these children.

Age 20: The brain weighs 1400 gm, and it represents the typical "adult" brain with active functioning of each of its structural components and related interconnections. The brain appears as a compact organ with obvious convolutions, or *gyri.* If the gyri were smoothed out, the flattened, spread-out brain would occupy approximately 2.5 square feet; the presence of gyri, and their adjacent *sulci* (or fissures), has helped reduce this space to one-third its size. The different structures of the adult brain are generally described according to its three major ontogenic subdivisions: the rhombencephalon, the mesencephalon, and the prosencephalon. Table 1.2 highlights the prominent structures at each level of the brain, while Figures 1.3 through 1.7 depict the location of the different structures.

After age 30, the brain loses .25 percent of its mass each year. The rate of shrinkage is influenced on lifestyle; for example, alcohol consumption has been hypothesized as a contributing factor because it is toxic to the brain. By age 80 there is approximately 7 percent reduction in brain weight (nearly 100 grams).

RHOMBENCEPHALON

The hollow core of the rhombencephalon is the *fourth (4th) ventricle,* which is a cavity filled with cerebrospinal fluid (CSF). Three structures define this lowest, posterior level of the brain: the medulla oblongata, pons, and cerebellum.

1. The medulla oblongata, abbreviated as the *medulla,* is the lowermost, or caudal region of the brain. It continues downward with the spinal cord, and appears bulgier than the spinal cord. It is composed of both gray and white matter to include the following structures:
   - *Cranial nerve (CN) nuclei,* are clusters of cells that give rise to the last four cranial nerves. For example, *nucleus ambiguous* forms the efferent fibers for cranial nerves IX (*glossopharyngeal*), X (*vagus*) and XI (*spinal accessory*), while cranial nerve XII (*hypoglossal*) originates from the *hypoglossal nucleus.*
   - The *reticular formation,* or *reticular activating system,* are groups of

Table 1.2. Structures Within the Three Primary Divisions of the Brain.

Rhombencephalon	Mesencephalon	Prosencephalon
Myelencephalon →	Corpora quadrigemina (superior & inferior colliculi)	*Diencephalon* →
Medulla oblongata (Medulla)	Red nucleus	Thalamus
Reticular formation	Substantia nigra	Hypothalamus (optic chiasm, hypophysis, infundibulum, mammillary body)
CN nuclei (IX, X, XI & XII)	Reticular formation	Epithalamus (pineal body, post commissure)
Inferior olivary nucleus	CN nuclei (III & IV)	Metathalamus (medial & lateral geniculates)
Vestibulocochlear nucleus	Cerebral peduncles (crus cerebri)	Subthalamus (subthalamic nucleus)
Ascending & descending (pyramids) tracts	Cerebral aqueduct	
		3rd ventricle
Metencephalon →		*Telencephalon* →
Pons		Right & left hemispheres (cerebral cortex)
Pontine nucleus		Five lobes (frontal, parietal, temporal, occipital, limbic)
Reticular formation		+
CN nuclei (V, VI & VII)		Corpus callosum
Ascending & descending tracts		+
+		Corpus striatum: basal ganglia (caudate, putamen & globus pallidus) + internal & external capsules
Cerebellum (2 hemispheres & vermis)		+
+		Rhinencephalon (olfactory bulb & tract; amygdala, anterior commissure)
Cerebellar peduncles (inferior, middle & superior)		
4th ventricle		Lateral ventricles (& septum pellucidum)

scattered cells and fibers that are responsible for arousing, or alerting the brain to incoming signals. They also send efferent fibers to regulate involuntary, or vegetative, behaviors relating to respiratory, cardiac and swallowing functions. For example, these cells regulate the rate and rhythm of heartbeat and respiratory cycles.

- The white matter is represented as bundles of nerve fibers or *tracts,* which are organized as either the *ascending* or *descending tracts.* Ascending tracts carry signals from the medulla to the pons and higher levels of brain; descending tracts originating from the cortex appear as a swelling called the *pyramid,* which crossover to the opposite side (or *decussate*) to send signals down from the medulla to the spinal cord. Another prominent bundle, the *inferior cerebellar peduncle,* connects the medulla to the cerebellum.
- A complex arrangement of cells, the *inferior olivary nucleus,* collects and shares signals between the spinal cord and the cerebellum.
- The *vestibulocochlear nucleus* is another collection of gray matter that receives input via the cranial nerve VIII (*vestibulocochlear nerve*). These afferent signals are shared with the cortex via the ascending tracts, and with the cerebellum via the inferior cerebellar peduncles. The vestibulocochlear nucleus also sends efferent signals to the ocular muscles via cranial nerves III, IV, and VI, as well as the spinal cord.

2. The pons is located above the medulla and sits anterior to the cerebellum; it is distinctly larger, or bulgier than the medulla. It is also composed of the following gray and white matter:
    - Three distinct clusters of cranial nerve nuclei, the *trigeminal, abducent,* and *facial,* receive and send signals via cranial nerves V, VI and VII, respectively.
    - The reticular formation, which perform functions similar to that within the medulla by alerting (activating) higher levels of the brain regarding incoming signals, and also regulating involuntary reflexive behaviors pertaining to the head region.
    - A small cluster of *pontine nuclei* receives input from the midbrain and share information with the cerebellum.
    - The white matter at the pontine level also includes the ascending and descending nerve tracts. The ascending tracts carry messages to the midbrain, and to the cerebellum via the *middle cerebellar*

peduncles; while the descending tracts take the signals down to the medulla and the spinal cord.

3. The cerebellum implies "little brain" because it appears as a diminutive version of the cerebral cortex. It is situated in the posterior fossa of the cranium and constitutes the largest part of the rhinencephalon. The cerebellum also contains gyri and sulci, has two *cerebellar hemispheres* joined by a median *vermis,* and its gray matter is also external to its white matter. It is second in size to the cerebral cortex and if flattened, it occupies roughly the same surface area as a single cerebral hemisphere; however, when folded with its gyri it takes up much less space. It includes the following prominent structures:

   • The gray matter of the cerebellum is organized as three layers: an external *molecular layer,* a middle *Purkinji cell layer,* and an internal *granular layer.* The cells in the Purkinji layer are one of the largest neurons in the nervous system, while the cerebellar granule cells are the smallest vertebrate neurons. The Purkinji layer collects input from the molecular and granular layers and shares this information with the brainstem.

   • There are four clusters of other gray matter within the cerebellum; the most prominent of these is the *dentate nucleus,* which sends efferent fibers to the brainstem via the *superior cerebellar peduncle.*

   • The cerebellar peduncles are white matter that developed from the embryonic alar lamina. They connect the cerebellum to the rest of the brain via three pairs of tracts, which include the inferior, middle and superior cerebellar peduncles.

In general, the cerebellum is associated with refining signals regarding body position, equilibrium and timing of body movements, and thus it regulates muscle tone, balance and coordination of body movements. In recent years it has been implicated in the processing of sensory information as well. Some of its involvements include making fine discrimination between the pitch of two tones, or judging the duration of a sound signal, or estimating the time interval between two consecutive sounds. These findings, as well as problems relating to spatial reasoning, memory, attention, planning and impulsivity have been observed in patients with cerebellar damage (Bower & Parsons, 2003).

MESENCEPHALON

The midbrain is the smallest division of the brain, measuring about 0.8 inch (2 cm) in length. It connects the pons and the cerebellum to the prosencephalon. It is composed of the following structures:

- Cranial nerve nuclei for *occulomotor* (III) and *trochlear* (IV) cranial nerves.
- The *corpora quadrigemina,* which is a collection of four pea-shaped bodies of cells located in its *tectum* (posterior roof). The top pair, the *superior colliculi,* relays visual signals to the thalamus and they also are responsible for regulating visual reflexive behaviors. The lower, *inferior colliculi* relays auditory impulses to the thalamus, and they regulate auditory startle responses.
- Within its interior, the *red nucleus* is seen as a rounded cluster of cells with a reddish hue due to its vascularity and iron-containing pigmentation in its cytoplasm. It plays an active role in transmitting motor signals from the cortex, basal ganglia, and the cerebellum.
- The *substantia nigra* appears as a spotted cluster because of the melanin pigment in their cytoplasm. These cells produce dopamine that is consumed by numerous cells particularly those in the basal ganglia, hypothalamus, and the cerebral cortex.
- The *reticular formation,* although smaller in size, also performs the same functions as those at the levels of pons and medulla.
- The white matter at the level of the midbrain is more tightly packed than those at the level of the pons and medulla. These bundles of ascending and descending tracts evolved from the embryonic basal lamina and they are collectively labeled *cerebral peduncles.* The anterior group of these fibers represents the descending tracts and they are called *crus cerebri.*
- The hollow core of the midbrain is a thin pipeline, the *cerebral aqueduct* (or "aqueduct of Sylvius") carries CSF down to the fourth ventricle in the rhombencephalon.

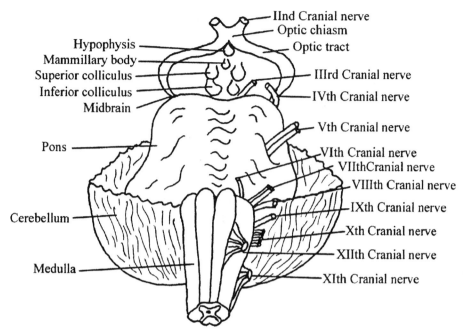

Figure 1.3. Anterior view of the brainstem structures.

PROSENCEPHALON

The two major subdivisions of the prosencephalon, or the forebrain, are the *diencephalon* (intermediate brain) and the *telencephalon* (end brain). The hollow central cavity of the diencephalon is the *third ventricle,* which also contains the cerebrospinal fluid. Otherwise, the diencephalon is primarily composed of several clusters of gray matter (see Figure 1.4):

- The *thalamus* is the most prominent egg-shaped mass situated on either side of the third ventricle. Because of their medial location, the two thalami are fused together in 70 percent of the adult brain. These groups of cells are responsible for maintaining consciousness, alertness and attention; in this respect they are analogous to the reticular formation in the mesencephalon and rhombencephalon. The thalamus also serves as the major afferent (incoming) relay station that forwards signals to the next higher level (telencephalon); it has been described to relay sensory-motor information to the cortex.

- The *hypothalamus* is located below and anterior to the thalamus, and extends from the optic chiasm to the mammillary bodies. This group of cells is responsible for regulating the primary drives such as hunger, thirst, reproduction, sleep and body homeostasis (temperature regulation); these cells also govern visceral and metabolic functions to create an individual's circadian rhythm. Extensive studies of the hypothalamus during the nineties have shown that it is distinctly larger in heterosexual men than in women and homosexual men. Some structures are considered extensions of the hypothalamus because of their proximity. One of them is the *optic chiasm,* which represents the crossover of optic nerve fibers to go to the contralateral (opposite) side of the brain. Another structure, the *hypo/neurophysis* (pituitary body) is a small pea-shaped body of cells that regulate the endocrine (hormone) secreting glands throughout the body. It is connected to the rest of the diencephalon by a hollow stalk called the *infundibulum.* Finally, the *mammillary bodies* are small clusters adjacent to the hypophysis, receive olfactory information from the hippocampus via the fornix.
- The *epithalamus* is located relatively posterior ward, and is a composite of several different structures. The *epiphysis cerebri* or *pineal gland* is a small cone-shaped cluster attached to the roof of the third ventricle near the superior colliculi (midbrain) and the posterior commissural fibers. Their exact function is unknown, but these cells possibly regulate endocrinal functions relating to reproductive cycles. Another cluster, the *habenular nucleus,* has connections with the amygdala and the hippocampus; it is believed to be involved in the integration of olfactory, visceral and motor information. The *posterior commissures* are fibers interconnecting the posterior sections of the two cerebral hemispheres.
- The *metathalamus,* also located posterior to the thalamus, is distinguished by two sets of cell clusters: the *medial geniculate body,* which relays auditory information from the inferior colliculi (in midbrain) to the temporal lobe of the cerebral cortex; and the *lateral geniculate body,* which relays visual information from the superior colliculi (in midbrain) to the occipital lobe of the cerebral cortex.
- The *subthalamus* is the final collection of cells located in front and below the thalamus. It contains the *subthalamic nucleus,* which plays an active part in muscle functions.

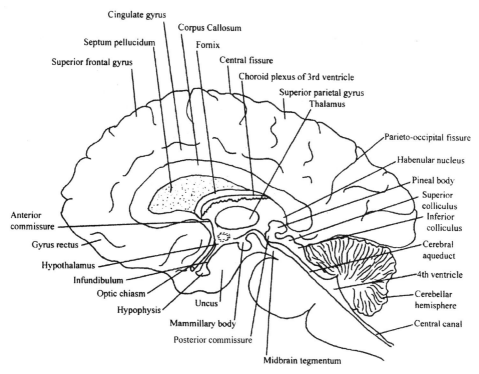

Figure 1.4. Medial view of the brain.

The final component of the prosencephalon, the telencephalon, is composed of two (right and left) *cerebral hemispheres,* each containing a *lateral ventricle* in its central core. The two lateral ventricles are completely separated from each other by a thin membrane called the *septum pellucidum.* The two cerebral hemispheres are separated from each other by the *longitudinal,* or *interhemispheric fissure.* This partition however, is not completed; they are interconnected by three bundles of white matter. One of these, the *corpus callosum* constitutes the largest and most prominent bundle of fibers to share information between the majority of the structures of the right and left hemispheres. Observations of female brains have shown them to have relatively larger corpus callosum, which has been attributed to their enhanced ability at reading emotions. The *anterior commissure* is a much smaller bundle of fibers that shares information between the anterior regions of the right and left hemispheres including the rhinencephalon. Finally, the *posterior commissure,* another small bundle inferior to the pineal gland, also shares information between the two diencephalon and the posterior regions of the two hemispheres (Figure 1.4).

The surface of each cerebral hemisphere, or *cerebral cortex,* is composed of *fissures* or *sulci* (grooves), and *gyri* or convolutions (ridges). Three distinct fissures have been used as references to establish the boundaries for dividing each hemisphere into distinct lobes. Two of the three fissures—*central* (or Rolandic) and *lateral* (or Sylvian) fissures, can be readily identified in a lateral view of the brain (see Figure 1.5). The third, *parieto-occipital fissure* can be seen in a medial section of the brain (see Figure 1.4). Each hemisphere also has several other fissures (for example, the precentral and postcentral fissures), which help determine approximate locations of prominent gyri within the different lobes. The three prominent fissures help describe four primary lobes, and a secondary lobe, within each hemisphere. The four primary lobes include the frontal, temporal, parietal and occipital lobes. The limbic lobe, including the insula, is considered the secondary lobe of the cortex.

The *frontal lobe,* the largest and anterior-most lobe, is bounded posteriorly by the central fissure and inferiorly by the lateral fissure. It comprises about 38 percent (range between 36–43) of the brain (Allen, Bruss & Damasio, 2004). Some of its prominent gyri, and respective functions, include:

- The *precentral gyrus,* also referred as the "primary motor strip" (4) is responsible for initiating the descending tracts that will carry information down to the lower levels of the CNS. This strip of cells control different muscles of our body that are under our volitional control, and sometimes their organization in the motor strip is depicted as the "homunculus" (see Figure 4.1, p. 68).

- The *inferior* and *middle frontal gyri* are situated perpendicular to the precentral gyrus. They control the voluntary muscle movements in the head and neck region that relate to facial expression, mouth, larynx, and pharynx. In the left hemisphere, the cells of these gyri also assume special functions that enable the act of speech production. For example, the posterior portion of the left inferior frontal gyrus, or *Broca's area,* is considered the motor speech area (44) because the cells in this region initiate the motor commands that regulate verbal speech. Similarly, the middle frontal gyrus of the left frontal lobe, or the cells surrounding Broca's area, is considered the secondary motor speech area (45 and 47).

- The *superior frontal gyrus* is also responsible for voluntary motor movements. In the left hemisphere the cells in this region regulate motor movements for handwriting or penmanship skills, and thus it is refereed as the writing, or "Exner's" area (8).

- The *prefrontal,* or orbital frontal, cortex represents the anterior most region of the frontal lobe (10 and 11). It is responsible for regulating executive functions such as reasoning, judgment, abstract thinking, self-monitoring, decision making, planning and pragmatic behaviors; it helps attend, target, and inhibit competing stimuli as well. Sometimes this region is considered the biological correlate of human intelligence and emotions.

The *parietal lobe* is located behind the frontal lobe; it represents 25 percent (range between 21–28) of the brain (Allen, et al., 2004). Its anterior boundary is the central fissure and its inferior boundary is the lateral fissure. Medially, the parieto-occipital fissure forms its posterior boundary to separate it from the occipital lobe. The primary gyri of the parietal lobe are as follows:

- The *postcentral gyrus,* or the "primary sensory strip" (3, 1, 2), receives somatosensory (touch, temperature and pain) sensations from the superficial and deep tissues of the body.
- The *superior* and *inferior parietal gyri* run perpendicular to the postcentral gyrus. They are responsible for integrating all incoming somatosensory signals with pertinent visual and auditory information. These cells are responsible for making appropriate recognition decisions that lead to cross-modality integration of information with previous sensory-motor experiences.

Two other gyri, the *supramarginal* and *angular gyri,* are located in the inferior parietal region near the posterior termination of the lateral fissure; however, they are not considered entirely in the parietal lobe. The supramarginal gyrus (40) surrounds the ascending limb of the lateral fissure, while the angular gyrus (39) surrounds the terminal limb of the lateral fissure. This region of the cortex has been recently coined the *TPO* (*temporal, parietal,* and *occipital*) junction because of its physical location relative to these three lobes. The TPO junction performs sophisticated cross modality integration such as color processing, and numerical computation including the concepts of sequencing and quantity; this determination has been made based on studies of individuals with synesthesia, who demonstrate the unique attribute of mixing up the five sensory signals. They are responsible for integrating all incoming somatosensory signals with related visual and auditory information. These cells are responsible for making appropriate (touch, taste, smell, hearing and vision) instead of keeping them independent of each other (Ramachandran & Hubbard, 2003). It appears therefore, that the convergence of different kinds of sensory and motor information, and the connections between the parietal and other lobes, implicates the parietal lobe for higher cognitive processing in humans.

The *temporal lobe* constitutes 22 percent (ranging between 19–24) of the hemisphere, and it is frequently referred as the auditory cortex (Allen et al., 2004). It sits below the parietal lobe, with the lateral fissure serving as its superior boundary and the parieto-occipital fissure as its posterior boundary. This lobe includes three prominent, horizontally situated gyri:

- The *superior temporal gyrus* includes a small *Heschl's gyrus,* which is buried within the Sylvian fissure. This gyrus is considered the "primary auditory cortex" where incoming auditory information from the medial geniculate body is first processed. Bordering the Heschl's gyrus is a relatively flat *planum temporale,* which can be barely seen in a lateral view at the lower edge of the Sylvian fissure. This region, embedded within the temporal, parietal and frontal operculi, is involved with secondary processing of sound signals; it is relatively well-developed in the left hemisphere. The posterior part of this gyrus in the left hemisphere is the *Wernicke's area* (21 & 22) for its special role in the comprehension of verbal messages delivered to the brain.
- The *middle* and *inferior temporal gyri* are considered as the "secondary auditory cortex" for their participation in making appropriate associations, and discriminations between different auditory signals.

The *occipital lobe* is the smallest and the posterior most of the four primary lobes; it constitutes about nine percent (range between 7–12) in relative proportion (Allen et al., 2004). Its anterior boundary is identified through the medially located parieto-occipital fissure. This lobe does not have any obvious gyri, however, it has a prominent calcarine fissure seen in a medial view, which runs almost horizontally to divide the occipital lobe medially into an upper and a lower half. The region surrounding the calcarine fissure is the "primary visual cortex" that receives all visual messages from the lateral geniculate body. The visual cortex is responsible for discriminating black-white, moving, fine details and colored stimuli.

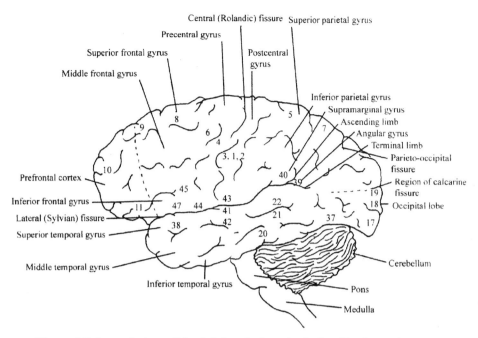

Figure 1.5. Lateral view of the left hemisphere including Brodmann's areas.

The *limbic lobe* (or central lobe, or island of Reil) is the central most, deepest region of the cortex. The term "limbus" implies that this lobe represents the border between the diencephalon and the neocortex. Phylogenetically, it represents one of the older parts of the brain; its cyto-architectural composition uniquely differentiates it from the rest of the neocortex. The limbic lobe is responsible for collecting new information, storing it as STM (short-term memory), editing or consolidating the stored information, and filing it permanently in other parts of the cortex. It also helps retrieve the stored data, and therefore acts as a two-way station for memory-related functions. The components of the limbic lobe include the ring of cortical tissue surrounding the corpus callosum (see Figure 1.4):

- The *insula,* or the *frontal, parietal,* and *temporal operculi,* represents portions of the inferior frontal, inferior parietal and superior temporal gyri that are embedded deep within the folds of the lateral fissure.
- The *cingulate gyrus,* or cingulum, encircles the upper regions of the corpus callosum and can be viewed in a medial section of the brain.

- The *fornix* is white matter embedded under the corpus callosum, and forms the roof of the lateral ventricles.
- The *hippocampus* resembles a sea horse and hence its name, is located along the floor of inferior horn of the lateral ventricle deeper to the parahippocampus, and is continuous with the fornix above. The hippocampus connects with several cortical and subcortical structures; one of its obvious pathways, the *locus ceruleus,* connects it between the midbrain and the prefrontal cortex. The hippocampus plays an important role in the formation and retrieval of both verbal and emotional memories (Teicher, 2002). Information must pass through the hippocampus before being recorded in the cerebral cortex. Research on hippocampus in animal models has revealed that rats exposed to chronic stress (6 months) show reduced hippocampal activity resembling decline in memory functions that is commonly associated with the normal aging process. Examination of the hippocampus from different birds species has shown that birds that store foods have nearly twice as large hippocampus than nonfood-storing birds; destruction of hippocampus in the food-storing birds has revealed that these birds continue to gather food but their ability to recover the stored food is impaired. Clinical reports of patients with hippocampal damage have shown that these individuals live in "eternal present," because they forget recent (short-term) events within approximately a ten-minute interval.
- The *uncus* is perhaps the most inferior portion of the limbic lobe; it is identified lateral to the optic chiasm, and can be best seen in an inferior view of the brain.
- The *amygdaloid nucleus,* or the *amygdala,* is an almond-shaped cluster of cells that is anatomically proximal to the basal ganglia deep within the medial region of the temporal lobe. Physiologically, it is linked with the limbic system, the rhinencephalon, and higher cortical functions. The amygdala is considered to be important in creating emotional memories.
- Two other structures, the *parahippocampal gyrus* located superficial to the hippocampus, and the adjacent *dentate gyrus,* are also components of the limbic lobe.

Other structures located in the interior of each cerebral hemisphere are the rhinencephalon and the corpus striatum. The *rhinencephalon,* or the "olfactory brain," is the early-formed part of the telencephalon.

This region is located below the frontal lobes toward the base of brain (see Figure 1.6). It includes the *olfactory bulbs,* which receive signals regarding the sense of smell via the first cranial (*olfactory*) nerve. The left and right olfactory bulbs are in communication with each other by a bundle of fibers called the *anterior commissures,* and they send signals to other parts of the telencephalon via the *olfactory tracts.* Other adjacent structures that also interact with the rhinencephalon are the amygdala and the hippocampus.

The *corpus striatum* (or corpora striata) represents an alternating arrangement of the grey and white matter, which gives this body a striped (striated) appearance, and hence the name corpus striatum. This region of the telencephalon is best viewed in a horizontal section of the brain (see Figure 1.7). Its gray matter is collectively called the *basal ganglia,* and they are responsible for organizing and refining the descending motor signals from the cortex and the cerebellum. The basal ganglia include three independent clusters of cells:

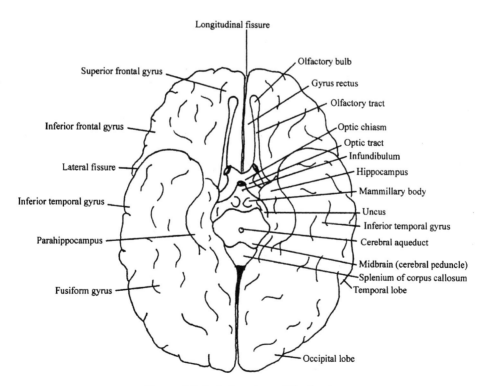

Figure 1.6. Inferior view of the brain.

- The *caudate nucleus,* located anterior-most, is perhaps the most prominent group of cells; its larger portion is its "head" while its "tail" is much smaller.
- The *globus pallidus* is found behind the caudate and lateral to the thalamus. Its degeneration has been associated with Parkinson's disease.
- The *putamen* is positioned lateral to the globus pallidus. The close proximity between the globus pallidus and the putamen sometimes make it difficult to differentiate them from each other, and therefore, they are sometimes collectively referred to as the *lentiform nucleus.*
- The *claustrum* is a thin sheet of gray matter that is lateral to the external capsule, but medial to the insula. Its exact function remains unknown.

The white matter of the corpus striatum is called the *internal* and *external capsules* because these fibers encapsulate the basal ganglia. The

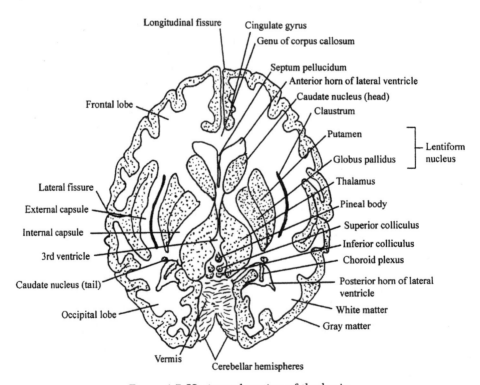

Figure 1.7. Horizontal section of the brain.

external capsule fibers form the lateral walls of the lentiform nuclei, while the internal capsule form their anterior and medial boundaries. These fibers constitute the ascending and descending tracts; they continue to ascend to the cortex as the optic and temporal radiations, or they descend downward as cerebral peduncles at the level of midbrain.

The concept of *limbic system* is much more comprehensive than the limbic lobe because it encompasses functions that incorporate several levels of the brain and the interconnections between them (see Figure 1.8). It links various cortical and subcortical structures such as the brainstem, diencephalon (thalamus, hypothalamus, epi- and subthalamus), the amygdala, and the cerebral cortex (five lobes). This phylogenetically oldest circuitry is responsible for fostering preservation and continuation of species through regulating feeding, aggression, reproduction, and other automatic behaviors which essentially integrate basic drives and learning.

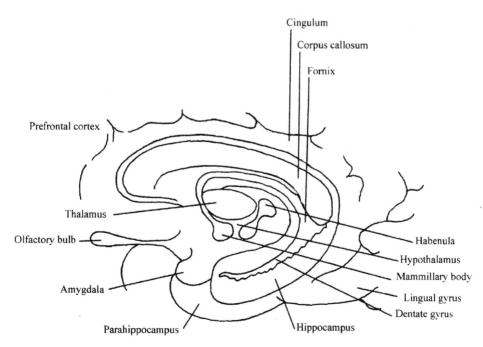

Figure 1.8. Some components of the limbic system.

SUMMARY

The different levels of the brain, their corresponding structures and locations reflect the fact that the simpler, and routine functions are handled by its lower levels. For example, the peripheral sensory organs serve as transducers that are responsible for changing some form of energy into electrical current, which is transmitted to the cortex with the help of the cranial nerves and their respective nuclei, as well as the reticular activating system, the rhombencephalon (pons and medulla) and the mesencephalon. These brainstem structures are responsible for accepting incoming sensory and motor signals, and also relaying motor and secretary messages from the brain to the different parts of the body. This level of the brain also controls reflexive behaviors pertaining to the head and neck region, as well as regulating homeostasis and visceral activities pertaining to respiratory, cardiovascular and digestive (including swallowing) systems. Furthermore, the rhombencephalon activates and conveys signals to the higher levels of the brain.

Although the cerebellum is a component of the rhombencephalon, its functions differ from pons and medulla. It integrates the visual and body positioning input, and connects with the basal ganglia to refine muscle movements for regulating body position, balance, and coordination.

The diencephalon (thalamus and metathalamus) receives signals from the lower levels, and prepares and distributes this information for the neocortex; in this respect, it is analogous to the reticular activating system for arousal and attention. The hypothalamus obviously regulates the cyclical functions of the basic drives. The subthalamus participates with the basal ganglia in refining motor movements.

Within the telencephalon, the rhinencephalon processes and stores olfactory information, while the basal ganglia organizes and refines voluntary muscle movements. The four primary lobes of the neocortex accomplish the final decoding (interpretation) of the incoming signals, as well as initiate the encoding (formulation) of complex behaviors. Each lobe processes and stores specific types of information; they also communicate with each other and with the lower levels of the brain. The cerebral cortex has the capacity to regulate, and override the operations of the lower levels by either inhibiting or accelerating their performances.

Finally, the limbic lobe is responsible for collecting and editing new and previously learned information; it stores new information for a brief period and distributes it for long-term storage. This lobe also helps retrieve new and previously learned (stored) information. In addition, the limbic system links the cortical and subcortical structures, and therefore, it integrates the activities pertaining to the primary drives to learning, self-preservation and continuation of species. It appears therefore, that although each level of the brain is responsible for some unique functions, they are interdependent through their complex connections with each other.

Chapter 2

BLOOD SUPPLY TO THE BRAIN

While the brain is credited to myriad and complex functions, it is refreshing to learn that it is composed of primarily (78%) water and some (22%) solid materials. The solids constitute proteins (40%), lipids (40–75%) and inorganic compounds. Water distribution in the brain is greater in the gray matter and in the intracellular environment. Although the brain shares two percent of body weight, it consumes 20 percent of total oxygen intake (or cardiac output). The principle source of energy for the brain is carbohydrates in the form of glucose. The necessary oxygen, nutrients and electrolytes are transported to the brain through blood, where it is converted to cerebrospinal fluid (CSF), which is then distributed and metabolized by the neural tissue. The brain utilizes each of its nutrients, electrolytes and oxygen, as well discards its metabolic waste, via the blood and CSF. It is important to develop some understanding of the blood flow and distribution to the brain because any disruption to its delivery has the potential for incurring brain damage. This chapter, therefore, describes the cerebral blood flow along with the formation and circulation of the CSF.

BLOOD CIRCULATION

Cerebral blood flow for young adults is 740ml (or 46 ml of oxygen) per minute. The brain maintains approximately 7cc of oxygen at all times, and it takes 10 seconds to consume this residual 7cc. There is a greater amount of blood flow to the gray than white matter. It is important to understand the delivery of blood to the brain because even a 4–6 minute vascular interruption can cause irreversible brain damage.

The blood supply to the brain is delivered by two sets of major arteries: the *internal carotid* and the *vertebral arteries.* These two arterial systems emerge from three major branches given off at the arch of the aorta just outside the heart (see Figure 2.1):

- The left subclavian artery helps gives off the left vertebral artery.
- The left common carotid artery divides into the left internal and external carotid arteries.
- The innominate (or brachiocephalic) artery angles toward the right side of the body to give off the right common carotid and subclavian arteries, each of which then divide as their counterparts on the left side.

The left and right internal carotid arteries mark the beginning of the *internal carotid system.* The internal carotid artery has a bulbous swelling at its point of origin (carotid sinus), which houses receptors that monitor any blood pressure changes to alert the brain to possible problems with blood flow. The two vertebral arteries in turn, form the origin of the *vertebral-basilar system* that will also supply blood to the brain. Both sets of internal carotid and the vertebral arteries travel upward toward the brain.

Each *internal carotid artery* arrives at the base of brain through the carotid foramen in the petrous portion of the temporal bone and via the cavernous sinus. Specifically, it enters the brain at the level of the midbrain between cranial nerves II and III, and lateral to the optic chiasm. At this juncture, each internal carotid artery gives off five distinct branches that form the primary arteries of the internal carotid system:

- The *opthalmic artery* supplies blood to the eyeball and ocular muscles, as well as the external frontal areas of the scalp and sinuses. It also connects with the ophthalmic branches originating from the external carotid artery, which is an important consideration when seeking donor vessels in vascular by-pass surgeries pertaining to the brain.
- The *anterior cerebral artery* is the anterior-most branch, which supplies blood to the anteromedial parts of the brain including the anterior and medial portions of the frontal lobe (prefrontal cortex), the parietal lobe, and parts of the limbic lobe (cingulum), internal capsule, and corpus callosum (see Figure 2.2). The two anterior cerebral arteries are interconnected by a small, bridging *anterior communicating artery.*

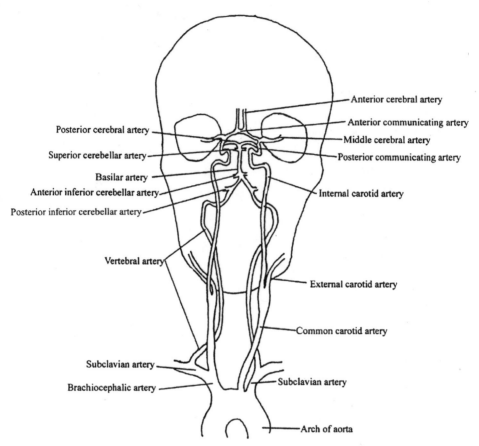

Figure 2.1. Anterior view of the major arteries that supply blood to the brain.

- The *anterior choroidal artery* supplies blood to the choroid plexus in the lateral ventricles. It also gives off small braches to the surrounding structures including the lentiform nucleus, hippocampus, and portions of the diencephalons including the thalamus.
- The *middle cerebral artery,* the largest of the cerebral arteries, courses upward to emerge to the lateral surface of the cortex via the lateral fissure. Its branches supply blood to most of the lateral surface of the brain including the three primary lobes (frontal, parietal and temporal) and the corpus striatum (parts of internal capsule and the basal ganglia). Specifically, it supplies blood to the middle and inferior frontal gyri, the pre- and postcentral gyri, the superior and inferior parietal gyri, the angular and supramarginal gyri, as well as the superior and middle temporal gyri; clinical-

ly, therefore, it serves the *perisylvian region* of the cortex (see Figure 2.3). This artery is significant not only because of its wide distribution area, but also because it is in direct line (or continuation) with internal carotid artery; this linear organization increases the vulnerability of the middle cerebral artery to possible vascular occlusions originating from the internal carotid artery.

- The *posterior communicating artery,* the posterior-most division, is a short artery that serves as a bridge to connect the internal carotid system to the posterior cerebral artery of the vertebral-basilar system. Its branches supply blood to the cerebral peduncles of the midbrain, the thalamus, optic tract, medial portion of the occipital lobe, and posterior portions of the internal capsule and corpus callosum.

The left and right *vertebral arteries* enter the CNS at the level of the sixth cervical vertebra through the transverse foramen, and ascend parallel to the spinal column to enter the posterior part of the brain via the foramen magnum. At this location each vertebral artery gives off three branches: the *anterior* and *posterior spinal arteries,* which distribute blood to the anterior and posterior parts of the medulla, respectively; and the third branch, the *posterior inferior cerebellar artery,* supplies blood to the posterior and inferior surfaces of the cerebellum. The two vertebral arteries unite at the upper level of medulla (or lower level of pons) to form a single *basilar artery;* the grouping of the vertebral, the basilar, and their respective branches, is also described as the *vertebral-basilar system* (see Figures 2.1 and 2.2).

The *basilar artery* gives off a series of branches on either side of the midline, along its upward ascent toward the cortex. Its lowest branches are the *anterior inferior cerebellar arteries,* which supply the anterior and inferior parts of the cerebellum, and the medulla. Next, several small *pontine* (or transverse) *arteries* leave its trunk to supply the pons. Another branch, the *labyrinthine* (or internal auditory) *artery,* goes to the inner ear. Above these branches, a pair of *superior cerebellar arteries* emerges to supply the superior surface of the cerebellum, pons and pineal gland. Finally, at the upper level of pons (or midbrain) the basilar artery divides into a pair of *posterior cerebral arteries* (see Figure 2.1).

The *posterior cerebral artery* is located at the medial and inferior surfaces of the temporal and occipital lobes (see Figure 2.2). It is linked with the internal carotid system via the posterior communicating artery. This artery supplies blood to the following inferior, posterior

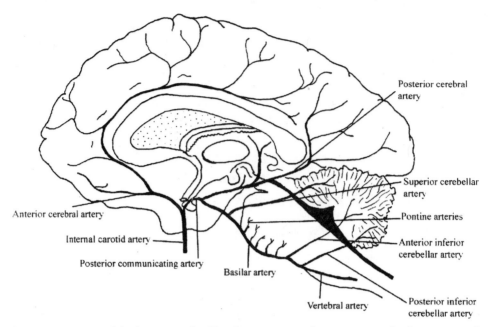

Figure 2.2. Areas of the brain supplied by the anterior and posterior cerebral arteries, and by the subcortical branches of the vertebral system.

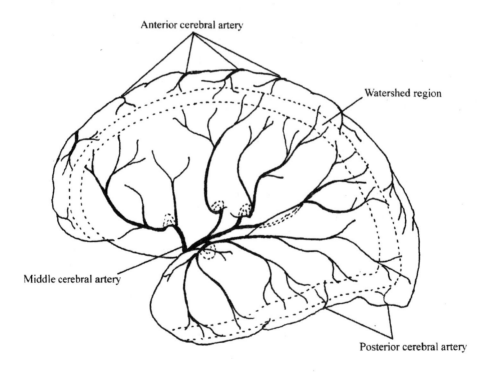

Figure 2.3. Blood circulation to the lateral surface of the brain via the middle cerebral artery.

Table 2.1. The Cerebral Arteries, Their Origins and Corresponding Distribution Areas in the Brain.

Vascular System	Arteries	Areas
Internal Carotid System	Opthalmic	Ocular & external frontal regions
	Anterior cerebral	Medial frontal & parietal regions; cingulum
	Anterior choroidal	Lateral ventricles; diencephalon; lentiform nucleus
	Middle cerebral	Lateral frontal, parietal & temporal lobes; corpus striatum
	Posterior communicating	Medial occipital region; midbrain; diencephalon; internal capsule & corpus callosum
(Vertebral)	Anterior spinal	Anterior region of medulla
	Posterior spinal	Posterior region of medulla
	Posterior inferior cerebellar	Posterior-inferior cerebellum & medulla; 4th ventricle
Vertebral-Basilar System		
(Basilar)	Anterior inferior cerebellar	Anterior-inferior cerebellum, medulla & pons
	Pontine	Pons
	Labyrinthine	Inner ear
	Superior cerebellar	Superior cerebellar & pontine regions; pineal body
	Posterior cerebral	Lateral & medial occipital regions; inferior-lateral & medial temporal regions; posterior-medial parietal region; diencephalon; midbrain; lentiform nucleus
	Posterior choroidal	Lateral & 3rd ventricles

and medial structures of the brain:
- The lateral and medial parts of the occipital lobe.
- The inferolateral and medial portions of the temporal lobe (inferior temporal gyrus and adjacent white matter, as well as the hippocampus and uncus).
- The posteromedial parts of the parietal lobe (superior parietal gyrus).
- The diencephalon (thalamus, medial geniculate bodies, pineal gland, hypothalamus, mammilary bodies and subthalamus)
- The midbrain (red nucleus and substantia nigra).
- The lentiform nucleus.
- The choroid plexus in lateral and third ventricles via the *posterior choroidal artery.*

The different cerebral arteries are sometimes clustered as two sets of arteries because of their distribution areas:
- The cortical, or circumferential arteries including the anterior, middle and posterior cerebral arteries.
- The central, or penetrating arteries such as the anterior and posterior choroidal arteries.

CIRCLE OF WILLIS

The blood flow between the internal carotid and the vertebral-basilar systems is shared through a circular arrangement of some of their blood vessels. This linkage, termed circle of Willis is therefore an interconnecting network of blood vessels is found at the base of the brain surrounding the optic chiasm (see Figure 2.4). Five different arteries make up the circle of Willis:
- Proximal parts of the two anterior cerebral arteries
- Proximal parts of the two middle cerebral arteries
- The anterior communicating artery
- The posterior communicating arteries
- Proximal parts of the two posterior cerebral arteries

The first four of these arteries are branches of the internal carotid system, while the last of the listed arteries comes from the vertebral-basilar system; variations in size of each of the participating arteries have been commonly reported. Numerous small arteries also arise from the circle of Willis to supply blood to the surrounding structures. The cir-

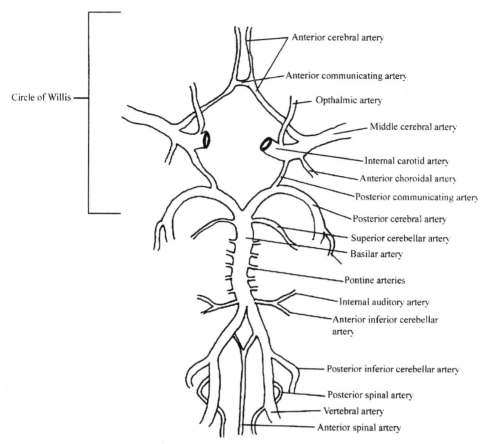

Figure 2.4. Arterial arrangement forming the circle of Willis at the base of the brain.

cle of Willis serves three important vascular functions:

- Helps equalize blood flow between the anterior and posterior regions **within** each hemisphere; this is accomplished with the help of the posterior communicating artery.
- Helps equalize blood flow **between** the two hemispheres with the help of the anterior communicating artery.
- Provides *anastomosis* (or joining) in case of blockage of either the internal carotid artery or the vertebral-basilar system. This concept is also described as *collateral circulation,* which refers to the provision of alternative supply if there is local obstruction. Four common points of collateral circulation are possible in the brain. First, the connection between the left and right internal carotid systems via the anterior communicating artery provides *interhemispheric anastomosis.* Next, the link between the internal carotid and

the vertebral-basilar systems via the posterior communicating artery provides *intrahemispheric anastomosis.* Third, the *retrograde flow* from the external carotid artery through the ophthalmic branch of the internal carotid artery helps support blood flow to the brain. Finally, the terminal branches of the three cerebral (anterior, middle and posterior) arteries provide *watershed anastomosis* to the regions overlapping the distribution areas of these arteries. The first two forms of collateral circulation are possible at the location of the circle of Willis (base of brain), while the latter two can occur above the circle of Willis (cortex).

The cerebral veins emerge from the neural tissue to pierce through the arachnoid and duramater, and they drain into the cranial venous sinuses. Unlike arteries, venous drainage is generally closer to external surface of the brain. In summary, blood circulation to, and from, the brain can be summarized through the following channels:

Arteries→Arterioles→Capillaries→Venules→Veins→Venous Sinuses

It takes eight seconds for blood to travel from the internal carotid artery to the jugular bulb.

VENTRICULAR SYSTEM (CSF CIRCULATION)

The ventricular system describes the formation and flow of CSF in the brain. Its key components are the four ventricles, or cavities filled with CSF located in the core of the brain, that evolved embryo logically from the neural canal. The size and shapes of the four ventricles vary to meet the CSF demands of the adjacent region and to accommodate the available space surrounding the neural tissue deep within the brain (see Figure 2.5). The description of each of the four ventricles is as follows:

- The first two ventricles are called the *lateral ventricles,* with one lateral ventricle in each cerebral hemisphere. They are the largest cavities situated in a horizontal 'Y,' or inverted 'C' shaped configuration; each is identified with a body and appendages termed the anterior, inferior and posterior horns. Each ventricle is medial to the frontal, parietal and temporal lobes, with the corpus callosum forming its roof and the thalamus at its base; laterally, each ventricle is surrounded by the basal ganglia. This relationship between the lateral ventricles and the adjacent structures can be seen in sagittal and horizontal sections of the brain (see Figures 1.4 and 1.7). The two lateral ventricles are completely separated from each other by a thin membrane called the *septum pellucidum.* Each ventricle contains an irregular-shaped membrane called the *choroid plexus,* which receives blood flow via the anterior choroidal artery (from internal carotid artery) to form the CSF. The CSF from each lateral ventricle flows downward into the third ventricle via a small opening called the *interventricular foramen* (or *foramen of Monroe*).

- The *third ventricle* is a single, midline cavity located in the region of diencephalon between the two thalami. It is smaller than the lateral ventricles and communicates with them via the interventricular foramen. The roof of the third ventricle is also lined with the choroid plexus, which helps form CSF from blood supplied by the posterior choroidal artery (branch of basilar artery). The CSF from this ventricle pours down into fourth ventricle via a thin three-fourth inch channel called the *cerebral aqueduct* (or *aqueduct of Sylvius*).

- The *fourth ventricle* is a diamond (or tent) shaped, much smaller midline cavity. It is located in front of the cerebellum and behind the pons and medulla. The choroids plexus in this ventricle is supplied by branches of the posterior inferior cerebellar artery. The CSF can flow from this cavity via two openings: median and lateral apertures. The *median aperture* (or *foramen of Magendie*) is larger and located medially at its floor; CSF flows from here downward to the *central canal* of the spinal cord. The two *lateral apertures* (or *foramen of Luschka*) extend laterally around the medulla to connect the fourth ventricle to the subarachnoid space.

Ultimately, the CSF from the central canal and the subarachnoid space pours out into the *arachnoid villa,* representing one-way openings that permit the discarded CSF to flow into the venous sinuses in the subdural space. From here, veins carry the deoxygenated blood down to the heart.

The choroid plexus needs some attention since it plays an important role in the formation of CSF. It is a specialized connective tissue that is embryologically developed from the ependymal tissue. This membranous tissue is located in the two lateral ventricles and in the roof of

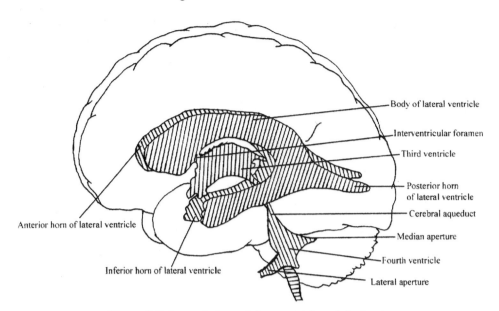

Figure 2.5. Lateral view of the ventricles of the brain.

the third (and sometimes the fourth) ventricles. The construction of the choroid plexus is such that it serves as a "sieve" to filter out cellular contents and other solid particles in the blood delivered by the anterior and posterior choroidal arteries. The outcome of this filtering system is the formation of CSF.

The CSF is a clear, colorless fluid bathing the brain, and it circulates in the ventricles, central canal and the subarachnoid space. It is composed of primarily water, glucose, electrolytes such as potassium (K^+), sodium (Na^+) and chloride (Cl^-) and traces of proteins; this composition is analogous to blood plasma. The brain contains an average 125 ml of CSF (100–140 ml range), of which, 7–30 ml (16–20 ml average) is found in the ventricles. Approximately 600–700 ml of CSF is formed per day; normally, CSF is replaced three times in a 24-hour period. The CSF serves several functions:

- It protects the CNS by cushioning it against any physical trauma from the surrounding bones.
- It provides buoyancy and supports the brain so that instead of its actual weight of 1300–1400 gm, the brain weighs only 60–70 gm when floating in CSF.
- The CSF supplies nutrition to the brain in the form of protein and glucose.

- It distributes energy in the form of electrolytes (K^+, Na^+ and Cl^-).
- By sieving off unwanted substances, it serves as an "ultrafiltrate" of blood.
- It removes waste products from neuronal metabolism from the brain.

The CSF pressure in brain is dependent on its rate of formation. The normal CSF pressure (60–150 mm of water) can be disrupted if there is blockage between the four ventricles, or if the rate of absorption of the CSF is altered due to any neurological anomaly. An example is *hydrocephalus,* which is the resultant clinical diagnosis due to excessive CSF accumulation in the brain. A couple types of hydrocephalic conditions have been described:

- A *communicating hydrocephalus* results when CSF is not adequately drained from the subarachnoid space into the venous sinuses. This condition has also been also referred as an *external hydrocephalus* because of the CSF accumulation in subarachnoid space.
- A *noncommunicating hydrocephalus* is determined if there is a blockage in the ventricles, or between the ventricles and the subarachnoid space. The term *internal* (or *obstructive*) *hydrocephalus* has been used in instances when CSF accumulates in the ventricle that is proximal to the blockage area.

Finally, the concept called *blood-brain barrier* is discussed with reference to the blood supply within the CNS. This concept implies that a "barrier" is created by cells lining the cerebral blood vessels, which restricts movement of specific substances. The blood-brain barrier allows some substances such as gases and water to permeate the CSF freely, and others such as glucose and electrolytes are allowed to pass at a slower rate; it is however, almost impermeable to larger molecules and proteins. This barrier, therefore, plays a major role in the selection and delivery of drugs for the management of a variety of neurological diseases.

SUMMARY

The functions and integrity of the different structures are dependent on adequate circulation of blood to the brain. The unique requirement of this organ that calls for conversion of arterial blood to CSF highlights the sensitivity and fragility of the neural tissue. Any variation or disruption to the normal circulation of blood or CSF can compromise one or more structures leading to their temporary or permanent demise. Such internal disturbances contribute toward the overt manifestations of clinical symptoms that define diseases of the nervous system.

Chapter 3

CELLULAR NEUROANATOMY
AND NEUROPHYSIOLOGY

This chapter reviews the microscopic structure and functions of the brain. It describes the cellular composition, their interconnections and activities that lead to the generation and transmission of electrical energy. Each of these cells is powered by neurochemicals that enable it to function as an elaborate processor. Some of these chemicals and their influence on brain activity are described in this chapter. It is essential to understand that these microscopic structures are constantly working whether the brain is consciously involved in making a decision or when it appears to be in a resting state. The intent of this chapter therefore, is to help appreciate the complexities underlying some of the overtly observed human behaviors, as well as the consequences of any adverse influence on the brain's habitual functions.

GRAY MATTER

The gray matter of the brain is composed of 100 billion cells represented by two broad groups of cells: the neuroglia and the neurons. The *neuroglia,* or *glial cells,* constitutes 80–90 percent of the cells in brain; they outnumber nerve cells nine to one. Neuroglia support, and provide nutrition to the neurons; these cells can also proliferate and develop into brain tumors. The glial cells also form the major part of the blood-brain barrier. Several types of glia have been identified throughout the nervous system:
* *Astrocytes* (or *astroglia*) are star-shaped glial cells that are generally larger in size and have many processes extending from their bod-

41

ies; they tend to concentrate closer to the neurons particularly in younger developing brains. Astrocytes contain the chemical "Nerve Growth Factor" (NGF), which is associated with brain development and learning; NGF has also been credited to the accelerated reorganization of the younger brain and its presence also explains the dramatic recovery in children following brain damage. Astrocytes tend to increase in number in an event of an infection, and this occurrence is called *gliosis.* An abnormal multiplication of astrocytes can lead to the development of a tumor, or *astrocytoma.*

- *Oligodendrocytes* (or oligodendroglia) are smaller-sized oval cells with fewer processes. They are primarily responsible for myelin formation in the CNS, and therefore, they are concentrated in the region of the white matter.
- *Microglia* are much smaller cells that are nonectodermal in origin (derived from mesoderm), supposedly brought in via blood. These cells have various forms; they are migratory and act as phagocytes (or scavengers) to remove infarcted (dead) tissue in the event of brain damage. Microglia also has the potential to convert to other types of neuroglia. As these cells age, they tend to accumulate high levels of beta-amyloid protein, which has been associated with Alzheimer's disease.
- *Ependymal cells* share the name with their embryonic origin. They form the inner linings of the ventricles and give rise to the choroid plexus.
- *Schwann cells* are the only glial cells that are not found in the brain. Like the oligodendrocytes, they produce myelin and are concentrated in the white matter; unlike the oligodendrocytes, however, Schwann cells are found in the PNS.

The number of glial cells decrease with aging, however, there is emerging evidence suggesting that the more one uses his/her cortex, the larger is the relative proportion of glial cells for the individual's age; therefore, one may assert that an active brain retards the aging process. Recent studies have established that glia influence the formation of synapses by either strengthening or weakening neural connections, and ultimately effect learning and long-term memories. Another indication is that glia also communicate with each other in a separate but parallel network (Fields, 2004).

The most important components of gray matter are *neurons,* or nerve cells, which are approximately two billion in number (10–20% of all cells) serving as the energy producers in the brain. Neurons convert chemical messages to electrical impulses and are somewhat analogous to a computer chip. The myth that only 10 percent of the neurons tend to be actively working at any given time is refuted by the fact that electrical stimulation of different areas of the brain has failed to identify any dormant areas. Although it has been established that mature neurons cannot multiply and are not capable of regeneration except in laboratory conditions, there is increasing evidence supporting the concept of *neurogenesis,* or regrowth of neurons in both animals and humans. Recent research has shown signs of neurogenesis in the olfactory bulb and in the hippocampus; also, successful migration of bone marrow stem cells to the brain and implantation of fetal tissue have shown signs of neurogenesis in adult human brain.

A typical neuron has a *soma* (or body) containing a *nucleus* and *cytoplasm* (see Figure 3.1). The nucleus and its nucleolus regulate the genetic and metabolic programming of the cell; their destruction will result in cell death. The cytoplasm contains several structures, one of which is *mitochondria,* which generate energy for the cell and control its metabolism; these small granular or rod-shaped structures are found in other types of cells as well. The *Nissl bodies* are large granular, protein-synthesizing substances responsible for the cell's metabolic activity; they are also involved in synthesis of neurotransmitters. The *Golgi apparatus* is a delicate network of fibers that are secretory in function; they produce and convert proteins from Nissl bodies to the axons. Another entity, *lysosomes,* serves as intracellular scavengers; they contain special enzymes that break down old or damaged proteins and lipids, and flush them out of the cell. The major inorganic compounds in the neuron's cytoplasm are the sodium (Na^+) and potassium (Ka^+) atoms in their ionic (or electrolyte) forms.

The neuron gives off projections, or arms, that are identified as follows:

- The *dendron,* or *dendrite* (plural form) are small branches that bring information to the soma; therefore, this region of the neuron is described as the dendritic, or *afferent zone* as well.
- The *axon,* or *nerve fiber,* is generally a single well-identified longer extension from the soma. It represents the transmitting, or *efferent zone* of the neuron since it carries the nerve impulse away from the soma; nerve fibers are collectively discussed as the white mat-

ter of the brain.
- The *axon hillock* is the location in the soma, devoid of Nissl bodies, from which the axon emerges; it also represents the region where incoming signals to the neuron are summed and it is from here that the nerve impulse leaves the soma.

Neurons have been segregated into different types based on either their anatomical, or biochemical characteristics. Anatomically, three types of neurons are identified (see Figure 3.1):

- *Multipolar* neurons, which have multiple dendrite and a single axon (e.g., pyramidal cells).

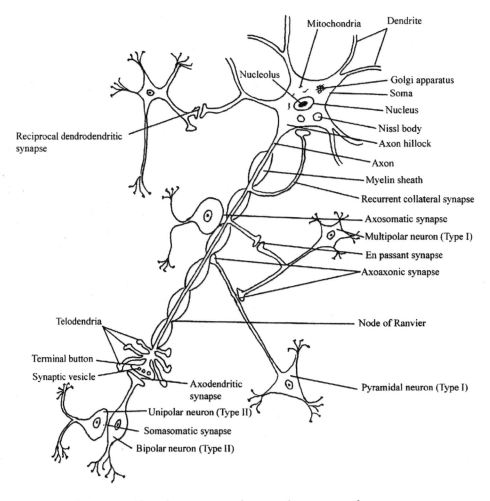

Figure 3.1. Neural structure and types of neurons and synapses.

- *Bipolar* neurons have a single dendron and an axon (e.g., granule cells).
- *Unipolar* neurons give off a single extension from the soma, which bifurcates at a short distance from the cell into an afferent (dendron) and an efferent (axon) zone (e.g., posterior root ganglion cell).

Neurons can also be differentiated according to their biochemical constitution whenever they are exposed to the Golgi stain; the cell's reaction to the stain has resulted in the identification of three types of neurons:

- *Golgi Type I cells* represent multipolar cells with multiple dendrite and long axons, which form the projection fibers and tracts in the brain. Examples include the *pyramidal* and *Purkinji cells.*
- *Golgi Type II cells* are unipolar and bipolar cells with short axons such as the *horizontal, stellate* (unipolar) and *granule cells,* which form short association fibers. These cells outnumber the type I cells, and they tend to be slower when responding to stimulation.
- *Golgi Type III cells* have no specific anatomical shape, but they do have long axons. Examples of cells in this group include the *Martinotti* and *fusiform* (conical shape) *cells.*

The rationale underlying the study of the cell type relates to the fact that it helps understand the cell's anatomical connections (linkage), as well as its physiological discharge pattern to activate different neural circuits. Typically, neurons arrange themselves in clusters; a single cluster of cells is called a *ganglion* or *ganglia* (plural form), or a *nucleus.*

Neurons are organized in six distinguishable layers in the cerebral cortex (gray matter). The relative thickness of each of these layers varies in different gyri. For example, the gray matter may be as thick as 4.5 cm in the precentral gyrus, but it may be reduced to 1.5 mm in the calcarine sulcus. This anatomical variation was used by Brodmann to identify different functional areas in the cortex. The six cellular layers are organized as follows (see Figure 3.2):

1. *Molecular layer* is the external-most layer composed primarily of Golgi type II cells, which constitute the stellate, horizontal or granule cells with short axons. These cells serve associative function indicating that they share information with adjacent cells or gyri.
2. *External granular layer* is composed of some small-sized pyramidal (type I) and granule (type II) cells; these cells receive information

from slightly distal areas and are, therefore, afferent in function.

3. *External pyramidal layer* is concentrated with pyramidal (type I) cells, which are arranged so that the superficial cells in this layer tend to be smaller than the deeper cells. A few Golgi type II and III cells are also identified in this layer. The cells in this layer are afferent and associative in function.

4. *Internal granular layer* contains primarily type II cells and some small pyramidal cells (type I). This layer receives afferent information primarily from the thalamus; it is also observed as well-developed in the prefrontal cortex.

5. *Internal pyramidal layer* is composed primarily of pyramidal cells (type I) and some of the largest cells can be found in this layer particularly in the precentral gyrus (primary motor strip). The cells from this layer help form projection fibers (e.g., pyramidal tract); their axons are efferent in function.

6. *Multiform* (or *Polymorphic*) layer is the deepest layer containing irregularly-shaped and a large variety of cells. The functions of these cells are variable: afferent, associative or efferent.

During embryonic development, the deepest cortical layers are developed first, and larger cells matured from smaller cells and they migrated outward to form the outer layers; thus the external/upper layers were the last to develop.

WHITE MATTER

The region of the white matter in the brain generally includes nerve fibers (axons), and they are found in different levels of the brain. As indicated in Chapter One, they are identified as ascending and descending tracts at the level of rhombencephalon, and as crus cerebri/cerebral peduncles in the midbrain; while in the telencephalon they are noted as internal and external capsules. Nerve fibers generally travel in collective bundles to link different structures. In the CNS such collection of fibers are identified as either *fasciculi* (*fasciculus* if singular) or *tracts;* their collective course in the PNS is referred as nerve. Physiologically, fibers may bring information to the brain and its higher levels (*afferent* and *ascending fibers,* respectively), or they may take information from the higher levels and out of the brain (*descending* and *efferent fibers*). Based on their location and direction, three major

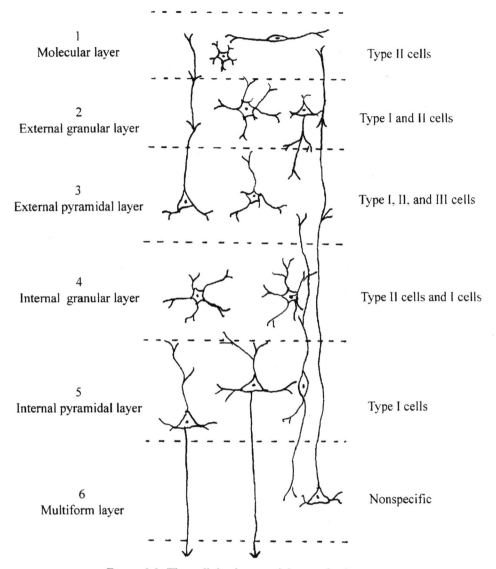

Figure 3.2. The cellular layers of the cerebral cortex.

groups of fibers are identified in the CNS:

- *Projection fibers* connect one level of the brain to another level; they are usually ipsilateral (or same side) in their path. Such fibers originate primarily from Golgi type I cells. These fibers, called *corona radiata,* are collectively arranged in a fan-shaped configuration to interconnect the cortex and the brainstem. The efferent projection tracts of the corona radiate from the cortex are the *pyramidal tracts;* while the prominent afferent projection tracts are the *thalamic projections/radiations,* which ascend from the thalamus to end in various cortical lobes (e.g., optic radiations).

- *Association fibers* interconnect adjacent gyri or lobes of the cortex. They are subdivided into two types: long and short association fibers. *Long association fibers* connect adjacent lobes within the same hemisphere and level of the cortex; *short association fibers* connect adjacent gyri to each other. The long association fibers originate from Golgi type I and III cells, while the short association fibers represent the axons from Golgi type II cells. Although specific examples of tracts representing the short association fibers is not possible due to their short length, several tracts of long association fibers have been identified in each hemisphere (see Figure 3.3). For example, the fan-shaped arrangement of fibers termed *arcuate fasciculus* interconnects all four primary lobes within a hemisphere. The *uncinate fasciculus* connects inferior and middle frontal lobe (F2 and F3 gyri) to superior temporal lobe (T1 gyrus). The *cingulate fasciculus* links the medial portions of the frontal and parietal lobes. The *inferior longitudinal fasciculus* forms the connection between the occipital lobe and the inferior parts of the temporal lobe; and the *superior longitudinal fasciculus* connects the occipital lobe to the parietal and frontal lobes.

- *Commissural fibers* interconnect corresponding regions of the two hemispheres; they are exclusively contralateral (opposite side) in their path. The *corpus callosum* is the most prominent commissural interconnection between the two hemispheres; these fibers are responsible for sharing information between corresponding regions of the two hemispheres. Other smaller bundles include the *anterior* and *posterior commissures,* which interconnect the anterior (olfactory bulbs) and posterior (hippocampi and diencephalon) regions of the two hemispheres, respectively.

The structure of a nerve fiber is analogous to a tree with the axon representing the main trunk; it can give off branches along its length, or *collaterals,* which connect the axon to adjacent fibers and neurons. Axons are the communication lines of the nervous system since they move the message-bearing electric impulses from one part to another. Sometimes the axon can send a *recurrent collateral* branch back to its own soma or dendron. At its distal end, the axon divides into multiple terminals, or *telodendria.* The final tip of each telodendron is button-

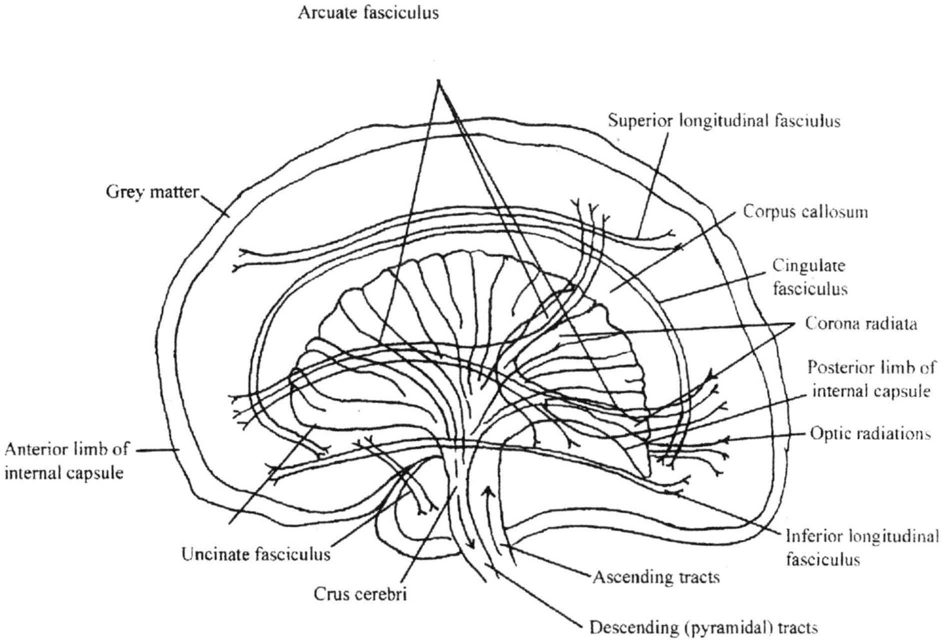

Arcuate fasciculus

Superior longitudinal fasciulus

Grey matter

Corpus callosum

Cingulate fasciculus

Corona radiata

Posterior limb of internal capsule

Optic radiations

Anterior limb of internal capsule

Inferior longitudinal fasciculus

Uncinate fasciculus

Crus cerebri

Ascending tracts

Descending (pyramidal) tracts

Figure 3.3. The projection and long association fibers of the brain.

shaped, and hence the name *terminal bouton* for this location. Within the terminal bouton are *synaptic vesicles,* which contain specific neuro-transmitters essential for brain function. The telodendron, or the terminal bouton, ultimately ends in the *pre-synaptic membrane,* which serves the distal boundary of the axon (see Figure 3.1).

Axons are tubular and uniform in diameter. They are frequently insulated by a protective sheath of white, translucent fatty tissue called *myelin;* such axons are therefore, referred as *myelinated,* or *medullated fibers.* In addition to its protective and insulatory functions, myelin also helps speed up conduction of the impulse. A bare axon may conduct a signal at 1–20 miles per hour, but one with myelin may conduct a signal at up to 270 miles per hour. Myelination begins about the middle of fetal life and is not completed in some tracts for up to 20 years. The oldest, first formed tracts tend to myelinate first, while newer tracts myelinate during the first and second postnatal years. Myelin is produced with the help of glial cells such as the oligodendrocytes (in CNS) and the Schwann cells (in PNS). Axons may show periodic breaks in myelin along its length called *nodes of Ranvier;* in such instances it is assumed that the axon is capable of *saltatory conduction,* which allows the nerve impulse to jump from one node to the next one to promote speedier transmission of the signal. Finally, an axon may have an outer casing, the *neurilemma sheath* that encases the myelin sheath (see Figure 3.1); this covering has been determined as an important prerequisite for regeneration of a damaged nerve fiber in the PNS.

NEURAL EXCITATION

All living tissues (cells) have residual electricity known as electric, or bioelectric, potential; the degree of electrical potential generated by a cell depends on the concentration and activity of the electrolytes in its vicinity. *Electrolytes* represent the ionic states of inorganic materials in the cell's cytoplasm (or intracellular) and outside the cell in the extra-cellular environment. The ions may be positively (+) (or *cation*) or neg-atively (–) (or *anion*) charged. Three of the different ions, Na^+ (sodium), K^+ (potassium) and Cl^- (chloride), are important to neuronal functions. Usually K^+ and Cl^- can move freely between the intracellular and extracellular medium via diffusion because the cell membrane is *per-meable* to these two ions. Sodium (Na+) ions however, are *impermeable* across the membrane during the cell's resting state. The disparity in the concentration of Na^+ ions within and outside the cell creates a dif-ferential potential measured across the cell membrane, which is termed *resting* (or *membrane*) *potential.* The recorded resting potential determines the cell's bias toward either the positive or negative volt-age, or *polarity;* typically the resting potential is approximately –80 mV.

Generally, neural communication originates when the cell's resting potential is altered due to either some stimulus. Any form of stimula-tion begins a series of chemical events that may ultimately generate an electrical voltage, an *action potential* (40 mV) or a *nerve impulse.* Behaviorally, action potential reflects the cell's response to the stimu-lation; action potential serves to excite other neurons and/or muscles and glands. The sequence of events proceeding the generation of an action potential is as follows (see Figure 3.4):

1. The cell is exposed to an *exogenous* (via the primary senses) or *endogenous* (inner thoughts, dreams) stimulation; this event dis-rupts the cell's resting potential.

2. The intra- and extracellular ionic movements are altered at the locus of stimulation, which enables the cell membrane to now become permeable to Na^+ and K^+. This free entrance to the positively charged ions has also been described as the activation of a theoretical "sodium-potassium pump." The increase in concentration of Na^+ and K^+ inside the cell is electrically reflected through the reversal of cell's polarity, or *depolarization*. This electrical event indicates that the resting potential has become less negative, or that the entry of Na^+ has changed the internal potential of the membrane from negative to positive voltage (less than -80 mV). The stage of depolarization reflects the subliminal effect of the stimulation on the cell, however, there is no overt behavioral manifestation that the cell has been stimulated.

3. Progressive increase in Na^+ and K^+ infiltration within the cell, due to the continual stimulation, is electrically recorded as the upward incline in voltage, or *graded potential*. If stimulation ceases during this phase, the sodium-potassium pumps stops, and the cell reverts to its resting potential because the voltage is below the cell's threshold; this characteristic of graded potential is considered a *reversible phenomenon*. Behaviorally, the observed chemical and electrical changes in the cell remain subliminal.

4. With continual stimulation, the graded potential continues to show an incline reflecting the infiltration of the positively charged ions ultimately resulting in the cell's saturation of these ions, indicating that the cell has reached its *threshold* (saturation point). This state is reflected as a sharp, positive electrical spike, or *action* (spike) *potential*, which is indeed the cell's response to the stimulation. Action potential is considered an *irreversible phenomenon*, also termed *all* or *none response* because its occurrence cannot be undone. Typically, action potential begins at the cell's axon hillock and spreads out along the axon in the form of a traveling wave of electrical activity. The time interval between the point of depolarization and the occurrence of the action potential is noted as the *chronaxy* or excitation time.

5. Occurrence of the action potential results in the cessation of the sodium-potassium pump, which marks the exodus of the positively charged ions from the cell so the cell can return to its resting potential. However, the cell may overcompensate by flushing out excessive Na^+ (or K^+) than necessary and reflect a downward dip

Extracellular space

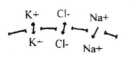

Cell cytoplasm (soma)

Resting state
(No stimulation)

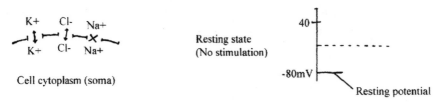

40

-80mV

Resting potential

K+   Cl-   Na+

K-   Cl-   Na+

Na+ channel opens

Onset of stimulation

40

-80mV

Depolarization

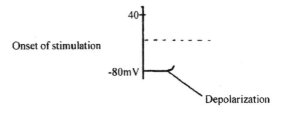

K+   Cl-   Na+

K+   Cl-   Na+

Continual stimulation

40

Threshold

-80mV

Graded potential

K+   Cl-   Na+

K+   Cl-   Na+

Na+ channel closes

Cellular response

40

Threshold

-80mV

Action potential

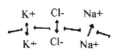

K+   Cl-   Na+

K+   Cl-   Na+

Return to resting state

40

Refractory period

-80mV

Hyperpolarization

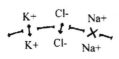

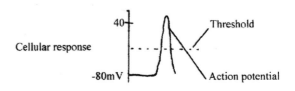

Figure 3.4. Biochemical (left side) and electrical (right side) events representing neuronal
stimulation and response.

toward the excessive negative polarity, or *hyperpolarization*. The cell promptly corrects this oversight and restores its resting potential.

The period following an action potential when no amount of stimulation will trigger a response (or action potential) is noted as the *absolute refractory period*. This interval is analogous to a resting, or recouping period for the cell to restore its chemical balance. The cell may shorten its refractory period, or demonstrate a *relative refractory period*, if the subsequent stimulation is stronger than the preceding stimulus. It is possible for a neuron to generate action potentials at a rate of 300 per second.

NEURAL TRANSMISSION

The sharing of information between neurons (or action potential propagation) occurs through two options. The traditional path of nerve conduction has been described through *synaptic transmission*. A *synapse* is a functional, or physiological, connection between the neurons; there is no structural joining between neurons and the linkage results from chemical mediators. Synapses can occur at different levels of CNS and PNS, and they are responsible for sharing neural signals between different structures. Synaptic activity is staggering; a typical cortical neuron may have up to 150,000 synapses through its dendrite and the different types of neurons in the CNS may average between 1,000 and 10,000 synapses. Synapses develop from neuronal demands during learning and growth; some synapses persist throughout life, while others may wither away from nonuse. Synaptic connections in the CNS can occur between different locations (see Figure 3.1):

- An *axodendritic synapse* can occur between an axon and the dendron of the connecting neuron.
- An *axosomatic synapse* can occur between an axon and the soma of the connecting neuron.
- An *axoaxonic synapse* can occur between two interconnecting axons.
- A *somasomatic synapse* can share information between two adjacent somas (cell bodies).
- An *en passant synapse* can occur between the collateral of one axon and another cell's axon, or it may occur between two adjacent collaterals as well.

- A *reciprocal dendrodendritic synapse* may occur between two dendrite (or dendron-to-dendron connection).

Three structural landmarks play an active role during synaptic transmission (see Figure 3.5). First component is the *presynaptic membrane* located at the distal end of the terminal bouton that is sending the action potential. The second component is the membrane of the receiving neuron, or the *postsynaptic membrane.* The extracellular space,

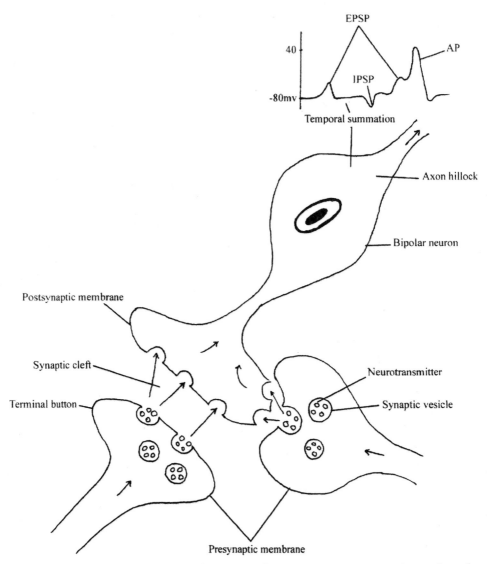

Figure 3.5. Structural components of synapse reflecting synaptic transmission and resultant temporal summation of excitatory (EPSP) and inhibitory (IPSP) postsynaptic potentials.

or *synaptic cleft,* between the pre-and postsynaptic membranes constitutes the final structural element.

The activation of the synapse occurs via chemical mediators known
as *neurotransmitters.* Neurotransmitters are special chemicals stored in
synaptic vesicles (containers) within the terminal boutons of the presynaptic membrane. Neurotransmitters are released from the synaptic
vesicles when an action potential arrives at the terminal bouton or the
presynaptic membrane; they cross the synaptic cleft to bind with the
postsynaptic membrane, thus leading to chemical changes at the postsynaptic membrane. Basically, neurotransmitters are responsible for
transmission of all nerve impulses throughout the nervous system.

It is speculated that there are about 200 different kinds of neurotransmitters in the CNS, and that more than 50 varieties of neurotransmitters may be involved in a typical synaptic activity in the brain.
Neurotransmitters may result in either an *excitatory* or an *inhibitory*
electrical potential across the postsynaptic membrane. Some neurotransmitters that are frequently discussed in neuroscience include the
following:

- *Acetylcholine* is the most common neurotransmitter found at all levels of the CNS and PNS; it generally creates an excitatory postsynaptic response. Its progressive deficiency in the CNS is associated with dementia of the Alzheimer's type, while its insufficiency in the PNS is associated with Myasthenia Gravis.
- *Epinephrine,* also classified as *catecholamine,* is found in both CNS
  and PNS and is also excitatory in effect. Its release is blocked by
  drugs called beta blockers to slow down an overactive sympathetic nervous system; such drugs are used to lower high blood
  pressure and prescribed to people who have experienced severely stressful experiences.
- *Norepinephrine,* also classified as catecholamine, is also found in
  both the CNS and the PNS. In the CNS, it is most active at the
  brainstem level for arousal and attention of the circuits, thus serving as a natural stimulant at this level of the brain. Its deficiency
  has been associated with symptoms of depression. A common
  synthetic version of norepinephrine is amphetamine.
- *Serotonin,* also known as 5-hydroxytryptamine or 5-HT, was first
  isolated in 1933 and given its current name in 1947. Serotonin is
  found only in the CNS; it is produced by the Raphe nuclei (midbrain) and is also concentrated at the brainstem. Foods high in

sugar and starch, as well as exercise tend to boost serotonin resulting in feelings of calmness and general improvement in mood.
Neural circuits that use norepinephrine and serotonin have connections between the hypophysis, the hypothalamus, amygdala,
hippocampus and the prefrontal cortex; this finding explains
abnormalities in sleep, hunger and metabolism associated with
their deficiency. Serotonin enhancing drugs, or antidepressants
manipulates serotonin level by blocking its "re-uptake," thus
allowing serotonin to remain in the synapse and interact with its
target postsynaptic membrane for a longer period. Serotonin
enhancers have also been found to encourage neurogenesis; in
children, however, these groups of antidepressants have shown to
induce suicidal and violent behaviors. Some synthetic equivalents
of serotonin enhancers such as cocaine and amphetamines produce short but intense euphoria, and they have been shown to
improve mood, energy, and focus. Their adverse affect however,
is vasoconstriction, which can induce a brain or heart attack.
Another drug, "Ecstasy" (or fenfluramine), does more than blocks
the re-uptake of residual serotonin; it also releases large amount of
serotonin resulting in brain damage from the excessive depletion.

- *Agiin* is also found primarily in the CNS. It is important for synaptic connections that are most active during the learning of new
  information. Its presence in the PNS has been restricted to the
  myoneural junction.
- *Nitric oxide* (NO) has been determined an important mediator in
  the release of excitatory neurotransmitters and in strengthening
  the synaptic connections. It plays a negative role, however, in
  triggering symptoms of migraine.
- *Dopamine,* found exclusively in the CNS, helps stimulate the feelings of pleasure and sense of well-being. Although found in both
  cortical and subcortical structures, dopamine is normally produced in the substantia nigra (midbrain), and conveyed to the
  basal ganglia where it helps regulate (inhibit) the descending
  motor impulses. Its deficiency, particularly in globus pallidus has
  been associated with Parkinson's disease. Shortage of dopamine
  receptors has also been associated with chronic, severe weight
  problems and addictive behaviors; its imbalance at the cortical
  level is associated with schizophrenia.
- *Glutamate,* known as brain's chemical kingpin of neural excitation,

also plays a dominant role in memory formation. It is found in the CNS and its deficiency is also associated with schizophrenia.

- *Gamma amino butyric acid* (GABA) is also found at all levels of the CNS. It is a derivative of glutamate, and it inhibits muscle movements. Its deficiency is linked with epilepsy and with Huntington's disease.

- *Glucocorticoids* are found in both the CNS and PNS. Within the CNS, they are concentrated in the limbic system particularly in the amygdala and locus ceruleus. They tend to have an inhibitory effect on neurogenesis but they have been known to have an excitatory effect as well.

- *Corticotropin-releasing hormone* (CRH) is found in the amygdala; its exact role is not known at present time.

- *Oxytocin,* produced in the limbic system, is absorbed by receptors in dopamine-rich region suggesting that it is linked with our reward ("feel good") circuitry. Its effects are heightened by estrogen and dampened by testosterone, which perhaps explains gender differences under stressful situations. Oxytocin helps develop, and regulate, social memory; its low level in individuals with autism perhaps explains their failure to form strong social bonds.

- *Peptides,* a distinct group of neurotransmitters also produced in the CNS, govern the excitatory and inhibitory effects of different neurotransmitters. Some examples include encephalins, endorphins and substance P. These chemicals can override the normal excitatory or inhibitory effects of neurotransmitters, and they are analogous to natural painkillers or antidepressants. For example, transcendental meditation has been found to help control pain because it enhances peptide activity. Peptides have been found to be elevated in children with autism, which may explain their ability to tolerate aversive self-stimulation behaviors for prolonged periods. A common example of synthetic peptides is morphine, which inhibits pain perception; another example, the chemical capsacum found in hot pepper, serves as a painkiller by blocking the brain's perception of pain signals.

Other neurochemicals in the brain have also been identified in recent years. One example is the protein called *Cyclic Adenosine Monophosphate Response Element Binding* (or CREB) found in the cell's nucleus; it plays an important role in the formation of long-term memory. Another protein, *Brain-Derived Neurotrophic Factor* (or BDNF) is found in the limbic system and seems to aid neurogenesis.

Synaptic transmission, or the transference of the action potential across the synapse, has been described through a series of events. First, the action potential (nerve impulse) arrives at the presynaptic membrane in the terminal bouton (see Figure 3.5). This event leads to the release of the neurotransmitters from the synaptic vesicles, and cross the synaptic cleft to bind with the postsynaptic membrane. As a result, the postsynaptic membrane loses it semipermeable characteristic, or its resting potential is disrupted. This disruption at the postsynaptic membrane can lead to depolarization if the binding neurotransmitter is excitatory in nature, or it can induce hyperpolarization if an inhibitory neurotransmitter is involved. The mediation of an excitatory neurotransmitter will be reflected in electrical changes that will proceed from depolarization to graded potential, and ultimately result in a localized *excitatory postsynaptic potential* (EPSP). The consequence of a mediating inhibitory neurotransmitter will show a progression from hyperpolarization to polarized graded potential, and end in local *inhibitory postsynaptic potential* (IPSP) (see Figure 3.5). The strength of the transmission is influenced by the amount of neurotransmitter released in the synaptic cleft, and how long the neurotransmitter remains there before its re-uptake in the synaptic vesicles. Sometimes *presynaptic inhibition* (inhibition without hyperpolarization) can occur from the influence of another axon, or its collateral, at the axon terminal, and reduce the amount of depolarization at the postsynaptic membrane. An example of presynaptic inhibition is the influence of touch on pain sensation where fibers conducting touch sensation can lower the perception of pain; this influence may explain the positive benefits of acupuncture.

Another form of neural conduction, *volume transmission,* has also been mentioned since the 1990s as an adjunct, or complementary, path for neural connections; it is not an alternative to synaptic transmission. Volume transmission is based on the premise that that neurochemicals travel through the extracellular medium, and that they can be detected by a remote cell of it shares the appropriate receptor; the outcome of such linkage is the activation of the remote receptor and resulting in an action potential at its cell. This concept is analogous to the release of a hormone from a peripheral gland into the bloodstream, which has the potential to affect cells remote from its point of origin. Recent information on glial communication endorses the presence and importance of volume transmission. Astrocytes utilize the *Adenosine Triphosphate* (or ATP) molecules that are normally released with neurotransmitters at the presynaptic membrane to send chemical signals to activate nearly glial cells through the extracellular environment. The activated astrocytes have the ultimate potential to either strengthen or weaken s synaptic connection (Fields, 2004). Such indirect interconnectivity between neurons and glia also help explain unpredicted improvement of functions in brain-damaged individuals.

NEURAL SUMMATION AND TYPES OF CIRCUITRY

All neurons are preprogrammed to add the incoming impulses; this prerequisite leads to the formation of action potentials. A single EPSP or IPSP is not strong enough to drive the postsynaptic membrane to its threshold, but series of EPSPs and IPSPs can be added together in a process called *summation*. Based on its structure, a neuron can sum the impulses via either *spatial summation* or *temporal summation*. The anatomical location for all temporal and spatial summation is the axon hillock.

Spatial summation is defined as the sum of electrical activity from different locations at a given instant in time; it can detect subtle changes in depolarization from each space. This type of summation generally occurs in multipolar cells where the axon hillock decides to create an action potential after reviewing all EPSPs and IPSPs from each of its multiple dendrite (or postsynaptic locations). Spatial summation operates under the principle that time is constant, but space/location of the incoming signals vary; therefore, the cell receives simultaneous inputs from several directions, and prepares a single output (action potential).

Temporal summation is the sum of electrical activity from a specific location across a time interval. In this instance, the number of impulses and the time period between impulses occurring at a single synapse are summed until the signals reach the cell's threshold. For example, successive EPSPs from a single source are summed to form an AP. Temporal summation generally occurs in uni- and bipolar cells (see Figure 3.5).

Once the impulse is summed at the axon hillock, it can transmit the AP utilizing several different types of circuits. One type of circuit, *divergent circuit,* occurs when the cell shares its action potential with several cells in its vicinity. For example, a signal communicating pain sensation may be shared with different areas and structures to result in several possible reactions such as localizing the target area, moving the discomforting area or crying because of the pain. Divergent circuits are made possible with uni- and bipolar cells. An alternative type, *convergent circuit,* results when multiple signals merge at a single location. For example, motor neurons may receive several types of input, which they will transmit via a select cranial nerve to a corresponding muscle. Sometimes a cell may employ *lateral inhibition* to sharpen its message (action potential); it can accomplish this goal by inhibiting the performance of adjacent cells. Another form of neural circuitry, *reverberating circuit,* is a self-propagating system between cells, which if activated, can discharge the signal for a long time until its operation is blocked by an external source. This type of circuitry perhaps explains the observation of repetitive behaviors in both normal and pathological conditions involving the brain.

Finally, the concept of *long-term potentiation* (LTP) needs to be explained in the context of neural circuits. LTP is the result of repeated stimulation of a set of neurons to strengthen their communication across their synapses. The concept of LTP is used to explain the formation of long-term memories.

SUMMARY

The human brain is so much more energy-efficient than a typical personal computer. Although the gray and white matter of the brain is described as separate entities, their intrinsic connections and interdependency are highlighted through the study of neuronal activity. Neurons create links to communicate with each other through their synapses and with the help of different neurotransmitters. The interplay of each of these microscopic mechanisms is reflected at the macro level through observation of brain function and human behavior. The brain customizes itself through its internal and external interactions the result of which is the formation of unique synaptic wiring in each individual. Grasping the intricacies of the cells, their ability to generate and transfer electrical energy, and sustain their functions through production and sharing of chemicals, is a fascinating discovery into understanding who and what we are as a species.

Chapter 4

CEREBRAL SPECIALIZATION AND AGING

The brain is a unique organ because of its capability to perform myriad functions. The clusters of gray matter at various levels of the brain, and the impact of their interconnections, have been studied across different species. Such investigations have introduced the concept of *encephalization* implying that during phylogenic development, functions that are important for a given species are assigned to the last developed structures of the cerebrum (encephalon). The human brain is three times larger than the brains of the great apes; this fact is used to allege that more complex animals have larger brains. In humans, the last developed cerebral cortex regulates the most complex behaviors of our species. This chapter provides a general understanding of the shared and esoteric functions of the two hemispheres, including those behaviors that impact communication as well. It also reviews structural and functional changes that are associated with biological aging to appreciate normal from pathological decline of the brain.

LATERALIZATION OF FUNCTIONS

The neocortex in humans has evolved to organize itself so that certain functions are ascribed to either the left or right hemisphere; this concept is termed as *cerebral lateralization*. Each hemisphere proceeds to further demarcate select areas for functional specialization, or *localization*. The concept of localization of functions is validated through observed anatomical asymmetry between the two cerebral hemispheres; such structural variations verify that specific gyri assume responsibility for unique functions. Some examples of anatomical dif-

ferences between the two hemispheres include the following features:
- The left hemisphere weighs more than the right one, which indicates that it has relatively more gray and white matter.
- The length of the brain, as measured from the frontal to occipital pole, shows that the left hemisphere is longer than the right one in infants, but in adults the right hemisphere is longer than the left one and it also protrudes out anteriorly.
- The lateral fissure in the left hemisphere is longer and better defined than in the right hemisphere.
- The left planum temporale area is more distinguished than the one on the right side.
- The left parietal operculum is also larger and deeper than the right one.
- The left lateral ventricle is larger than the right one.
- The cells in the primary visual cortex tend to be larger in the left hemisphere.
- The left pyramidal tract (in medulla) is larger and thicker than the right one.

Each of these anatomical differences has been attributed to the physiological/functional asymmetry between the two hemispheres; they also provide the bases for the concept of *cerebral dominancy*.

During the early twentieth century, Brodmann assigned the cerebral cortex into different numerical areas based on the morphological arrangement of its six cellular layers. Originally, he came up with nine morphologically distinct areas, which later evolved into 50 areas, and finally into 200 different areas. The relative size of specific areas within the cortex is governed by each individual's genetic make-up and experiences. Some commonly identified areas within the four primary lobes are illustrated in Figure 1.5.

COMMON FUNCTIONS OF BOTH HEMISPHERES

Both hemispheres are equally responsible for the following functions (see Table 4.1):
- Olfaction, which involves perception of odor is controlled by the areas described under rhinencephalon located at the base of the brain under the frontal lobe.
- *Vision* (sight) is regulated in the occipital lobe. Area 17 surround-

ing the calcarine fissure serves as the *primary visual area,* and area 18 represents the *secondary visual area;* these areas accomplish visual perceptual and associative functions.

- *Audition* relates to the perception of auditory (hearing) signals. This function is controlled by area 41, or the *primary auditory area* in the anterior part of the superior temporal gyrus (T1), also known as *Heschl's gyrus.* Area 42 in the middle temporal gyrus (T2) and area 37 in the inferior temporal gyrus (T3), serve as *auditory association areas.*

- *Somesthesia,* or the perception of somatosensory information regarding superficial touch, temperature and pain, is localized to areas 3, 1 and 2 (postcentral gyrus) in the parietal lobe; this gyrus is also called the *primary sensory area/cortex.* The remainder of the parietal cortex contributes as the *association cortex* for such sensory signals.

- *Stereognosis* is the ability to recognize objects via touch or feel exclusively. This function results from the integration of all forms of sensory input, which is regulated by the superior and inferior parietal gyri.

- *Voluntary motor movements* are possible through the cells in area 4 (precentral gyrus), also referred as the *primary motor area/cortex* in the frontal lobe.

- *Executive functions* include the ability to abstract information, problem solve, reason, and make appropriate logical judgments and decisions. These functions are integrated in the prefrontal cortex, which includes the orbital and anterior portions of superior (F1), middle (F2) and inferior (F3) frontal gyri. The importance of these cognitive functions account for the relatively larger proportion of brain (38%) devoted to the frontal lobe. The prefrontal cortex has extensive connections with several subcortical and cortical structures, which enables this region to play a major role in the performance of several types of cognitive functions.

Typically, one hemisphere controls each of the above-mentioned functions on the opposite side of the body; such *contralateral* innervation results because 96 percent of the descending fibers in the brain *decussate* (or cross over) to the opposite side before they leave the brain.

Table 4.1. Functional Organization of the Two Cerebral
Hemispheres and Possible Disorders from Lesions.

Right Hemisphere	Left Hemisphere	Disorder
Olfaction	Olfaction	–
Vision	Vision	Blindness
Audition	Audition	Hearing loss
Somesthesia	Somesthesia	–
Stereognosis	Stereognosis	Astereognosia
Voluntary motor movement	Voluntary motor movement	Paralysis
Executive functions	Executive functions	Cognitive problems
Word retrieval	Word retrieval	Anomia
Visual spatial discrimination	–	Visual agnosia
Visual construction	–	Visual agnosia
Nonverbal ideation	–	Cognitive problem
Facial discrimination	–	Prosopagnosia
Tonal discrimination	–	Amusia
Metalinguistic ability	–	Cognitive problem
–	Fine motor coordination	Impaired dexteriy
–	Language production	Broca's aphasia
–	Language comprehension	Wernicke's aphasia
–	Reading	Alexia
–	Writing	Agraphia

SPECIAL FUNCTIONS OF RIGHT HEMISPHERE

The brain is also responsible for other functions, some of which are primarily controlled by the right or the left hemisphere. For example, both hemispheres can receive stimulation and make output decisions, but some of these acts are governed by one hemisphere. This implies that one of the two hemispheres can integrate, or override, the decisions of the contralateral hemisphere by assuming a "dominant" role during select functions. Although there is no obvious explanation as to how each hemisphere assumed the principle responsibility for select functions, their differential roles in humans are highlighted whenever there is damage to select areas of the brain.

The right hemisphere is primarily responsible for the following functions (see Table 4.1):

- Integration of visual signals in activities requiring perception, discrimination and judgment; this includes *visuospatial discrimination* and *orientation,* as well as visual organization of objects in space (or *visual construction*). Some common behaviors reflecting the integrity of these functions is seen through our ability to move around without bumping into objects, the awareness of our body in space, making quick and accurate visual discrimination between objects and shapes, constructing three-dimensional block designs, and the ability to distinguish and establish relationships between primary and background figures (objects). Impaired ability to accomplish these skills is generally identified as *visual agnosia.*

- *Nonverbal ideation* implies the ability to create unique forms of artwork such as drawing, painting, or a musical score, as well as literary creations such as poetry and fiction.

- *Facial discrimination* refers to the ability to recognize faces and facial expressions. It remains unclear if this ability relates to recognizing specific facial characteristics, or if it pertains to recognizing familiar faces based on previous experiences and learning. An impairment of this unique visual perceptual ability is called *prosopagnosia.*

- *Tonal discrimination* involves interpretation and use of speech rhythm, which includes detection and use of the suprasegmental features of speech including pitch, melody and rhythm. The term *amusia* is used to denote impairment in this auditory perceptual ability. It is important to note that tonal discrimination should not be confused with musical discrimination ability or the acquisition of a musical gift.

- *Metalinguistic ability* involves detection and interpretation of humor and metaphor. This complex cognitive skill requires integration of memory, logic, as well as sensory and emotional experiences.

- *Language comprehension* and *production* in approximately two percent of the population who depend on right hemisphere for the majority of communication acts; such individuals acquire *aphasia* if they incur a right hemisphere damage.

SPECIAL FUNCTIONS OF LEFT HEMISPHERE

The left hemisphere is also credited with several unique functions. One of these skills is *fine-motor coordination,* which requires integration of visual information during motor acts that call for details and precision. An obvious example is the need for eye-hand coordination during writing, which is reflected through penmanship; other examples include the proficiency in use of a variety of hand tools (see Table 4.1).

The most important contribution of the left hemisphere is *language comprehension* and *production* in the majority (98%) of the population. This fact is established through the prevalence of breakdown in language functions, or presence of *aphasia,* in individuals with left hemisphere lesions. Both hemispheres can produce sounds, but only the left hemisphere is capable of processing and generating meaningful verbal speech. Although deaf individuals, who use the American Sign Language (ASL), rely on visuospatial cues, they also process ASL signs in the left hemisphere; this finding is affirmed from their sign repetition performances, and from clinical reports of breakdown in ASL use subsequent to a left hemisphere lesion.

Historically, Franz Joseph Gall, an anatomist, was the first to contend that different aspects of language functions are localized to specific areas in the left hemisphere. This assertion was verified in 1868, when Paul Broca who was a French anthropologist, surgeon and neurologist, demonstrated from a postmortem report that the "motor speech" area was localized in the posterior part of the left inferior frontal gyrus. This area was determined to help formulate verbal speech and therefore, termed *Broca's area.* Six years following Broca's disclosure, Carl Wernicke, a German neurologist, identified the "sensory speech" area in the posterior portion of the left superior temporal gyrus, and thus *Wernicke's area* was coined in the literature. Because several areas contribute to language they have been grouped together into three zones (Benson & Ardilla, 1996):

- An *anterior* or *frontal zone,* which includes anterior portions of the insula (frontal operculum), posterior part of the inferior frontal gyrus (Broca's area in F3), and surrounding areas such as the foot of the middle frontal gyrus (F2).

- The *inferior,* or *temporal zone,* includes the posterior regions of superior (Wernicke's area in T1) and middle temporal (T2) gyri.
- The *posterior,* or *parietal zone,* includes the angular and supramarginal gyri.

Collectively, these three zones surround the lateral fissure and therefore, the term *perisylvian* is often used when reporting extensive lesions of the left hemisphere associated with aphasia. The middle cerebral artery supplies blood to the three language zones and therefore, its dysfunction contributes to the development of aphasia.

Verbal communication requires the cooperation of several cortical areas. For instance, the act of listening involves the primary auditory cortex which shares the perceived signal to Wernicke's area for comprehension. In order to speak, or respond to a message, Wernicke's area sends the decoded message to Broca's area which in turn, collects details from the association cortex and proceeds to formulate the outgoing message the outcome of which is sent to the primary motor cortex to project the signal out of the brain, and the ultimate result is moving the muscles (lips, tongue and larynx) for speech production. In case the incoming signal is visual in nature (written words), the visual cortex performs the first stage of decoding and then relays the message to Wernicke's area and association cortex for comprehension; the message is forwarded to Broca's area if it calls for a spoken response. The pathways for each of these acts are illustrated in Figure 4.1. Details regarding these language-related functions and their respective cortical areas are described as follows:

- *Motor speech (language production) area,* or area 44 representing *Broca's area* in the posterior part of the inferior frontal gyrus (F3), is responsible for initiating signals for speech production. Damage to this area is reflected as a language production problem, also referred as *Broca's aphasia.*
- *Supplementary motor speech area* includes area 45 in the posterior region of the middle frontal gyrus (F2) adjacent to Broca's area.
- *Programming/sequencing of speech syllables* has been associated with the left frontal insula (approximately 1 cm. wide beneath the precentral gyrus) based on CT and MRI scans of individuals with left CVA who have verbal apraxia (Dronker, 1997).
- *Exner's area,* or writing center described as areas 8 and 9 in the superior frontal gyrus (F1) controls hand and finger movements

for penmanship skills required for legible writing.
- *Language comprehension* is processed in area 22 or *Wernicke's area* in the posterior part of superior temporal gyrus (T1). This area is responsible for the interpretation of spoken language; damage to this area results in language (auditory) comprehension problem, or *Wernicke's aphasia.*
- *Word retrieval* ability involves activation of multiple areas including areas 39 and 40 representing the angular and supramarginal gyri, and area 37 (auditory association area) in the inferior temporal gyrus (T3). Word retrieval process involves activation of the previously described TPO junction for searching and integrating all sensory associations to help recall a target word or lexicon. Damage to this region may result in several possible impairments: *anomia* (or naming difficulty), *alexia* (or reading disturbance), or *agraphia* (writing problem).

The left hemisphere is considered the *dominant,* or major hemisphere not only because it is relatively larger, but also because it is responsible for the last evolved, most complex and unique (speech-

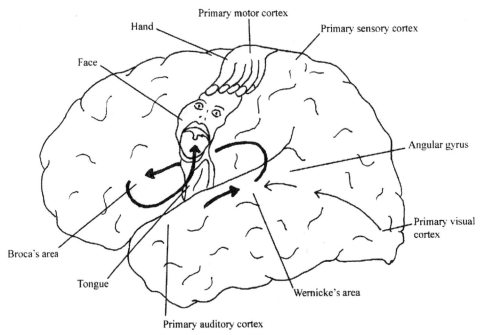

Figure 4.1. A simplified explanation of the primary cortical connections underlying the acts of listening-speaking (dark lines) and reading-speaking (all lines).

language) ability of humans. Although bilateral representation for voice and oral motor movements exist, their organization and synthesis for verbal communication are regulated by a single hemisphere, which assumes dominancy for this function.

Support for left hemisphere dominancy for language functions has been established through autopsy and clinical reports correlating left hemisphere damage and presence of aphasia. Studies on electrical stimulation of the cortex during the 1950s, and sodium amytol injections to the internal carotid artery in the 1960s, demonstrate speech disruption in normal adults whenever the left hemisphere was the locus of stimulation or the injection. In the 1970s two genes determining cerebral dominancy were identified; this finding explains why left-handed people are not always right-hemisphere dominant, and why they refute the traditional contention of a contralateral relationship between preferred handedness and the language-dominant hemisphere. Furthermore, ultrasound studies indicate that 92 percent of fetuses tend to use the right thumb when sucking; this observation supports the genetic basis for acquisition of preferred handedness that is independent of language functions. Finally, recent studies have linked mutation of a gene (FoxP2) on chromosome 7 to affect speech and language functions.

The association between cerebral dominancy for language and hand preference has resulted from a couple perspectives. First, hand preference and communication are considered complex traits that are observed only in primates and in humans. The fact that primates use gestural communication via hand movements perhaps serves as a foundation for this connection. However, use of speech as a mode of communication is unique to humans; this act calls for special cortical circuits, which explains the evolutionary separation of hand preference and language lateralization. This contention is corroborated through the observation that the majority of both right (95 to 99%) and left-handers (50–70%) show left-hemisphere dominancy for language functions. Some left handers (20–30%) however, demonstrate right-hemisphere dominancy, and few (approximately 15%) of these individuals demonstrate bilateral hemisphere representation for language as well.

Those individuals who demonstrate an ipsilateral relationship between preferred handedness and language dominant side, and who later acquire a language disorder are clinically referred to have *crossed aphasia.* Crossed aphasia may occur in either a left-handed person with a left hemisphere lesion, or in a right-handed person with right hemisphere lesion. The incidence of crossed aphasia has been reported to range between 0.4 to 2.0 percent; and the causes for the brain damage in such instances have been vascular and traumatic lesions, as well as tumors.

GENDER DIFFERENCES

Recently, there is some interest in determining a possible relationship between gender and cerebral asymmetry. Variations in brain size and structures are considered to reflect their relative importance to different animals. Studies of birds have shown that males have larger song control areas than female birds, and that male birds show a decline in size of the song control area between spring (mating) and summer seasons. The difference in brain volume between men and women is approximately a 100 c.c. Men tend to have relatively larger head size, higher proportion of white matter and CSF (ratio of 1.35 versus 1.26), while women have a higher proportion of grey matter. The frontal cortex and the limbic cortex (including the hippocampus) are bulkier in women than in men. On the other hand, parts of the parietal cortex and the amygdala are larger in men than in women. Analysis of cadaveric cells from the anterior hypothalamus has revealed similar size cells in women and in homosexual men, and that these two groups of individuals had smaller cell sizes than in heterosexual men.

Physiologically, the two genders show differences in performances for visual spatial and verbal memory tasks; men perform better on visual spatial tasks and women show superiority for verbal tasks. The brains of the two genders also respond differently to identical emotional memories. This is evidenced through increased activity in right amygdala in men, while women show greater activity in the left amygdala; these findings have been derived from analysis of evoked (spike) potentials at 300 milliseconds (P300) following stimulus exposure. Contemporary reports also indicate that the average serotonin production 52 percent higher in men than in women; this difference has been used as a possible explanation for the greater vulnerability of women to depression (Allen et al., 2004; Cahill, 2005).

AGE-RELATED CHANGES

Biological aging is a fact and its effect is also reflected in the nervous system. Some of the observed neurological changes are anatomical and physiological, and they are intertwined with individual life style as well.

One of the gross structural changes in the brain relate to the reduction in its weight. After age 30, the brain loses .25 percent mass each year; and by age 80, the brain has lost 7 percent (100 gm) of its weight. Other changes are reflected through shrinkage of gyri, widening of sulci, and some thickening of the meninges. Hippocampal maturation occurs earlier in life, during the first few months. In contrast, the neocortex, which is responsible for developing long-term memory, does not show signs of maturation until preschool years. These events explain why most adults cannot remember events that occurred before 3 to 4 years of age. Changes are also observed at the cellular level. For example, there is a progressive reduction in number of cells with rate of reduction varying in different areas of the brain; the greatest neuronal loss is seen in the frontal lobe, superior temporal lobe, and in the occipital lobe. It is established that normal cell repair occurs with the help of *telomeres* found at the tips of chromosomes; with successive cell divisions telomeres become progressively shorter until they cannot divide and consequently, contribute to cell loss. Cellular senescence has also been linked to increased arterial plaque formation that characterizes atherosclerosis. Older brains also show the formation of neuritic plaques and the appearance of neurofibrillary tangles particularly in the hippocampus.

An important contributing factor influencing the rate of change is alcohol consumption at any age. Traditional contention that the younger brain is more resilient than the adult brain has been challenged based on the observation that young brains are more susceptible to brain damage from alcohol consumption. The ill effects of heavy drinking are seen particularly in the hippocampus and the prefrontal cortex; this finding is of concern since these regions are important for learning, memory formation, and executive functions (Wuethrich, 2001). Another reported factor is gender; male brains have been observed to shrink faster than female brains however, no specific explanation is available for this anomaly.

Physiological changes in brain result from several factors, one of which is chemical changes such as reduced production/availability of neurotransmitter-related compounds. Within the cell cytoplasm, *ribosomes* (protein synthesizers) and Nissl bodies decrease in number. Also seen are changes in the arrangement of protein enzymes in cell cytoplasm; older enzymes go through gradual unfolding of these enzymes. Another obvious occurrence is the accumulation of *lipofuscin* (pigmented material) in cell cytoplasm. In addition, abnormal filaments are observed around the nucleus and Golgi apparatus; the excessive accumulation of such compounds is typically found in Alzheimer's disease. Mitochondrial mutations are also associated with the aging process and they underlie some of the neurological diseases among the elderly. Receptively, fewer stimuli are recognized implying that there is less arousal of neural tissue and consequently, fewer responses are generated. In addition, changes in synaptic potential also occur, which lower excitation threshold and lead to "blurring" of impulses. The progressive degeneration in myelin, seen around age 60, also impedes the efficiency of nerve conduction. Finally, vascular changes also contribute to aging. For example, reduction in blood flow exacerbates the decline in brain metabolic functions. Also, even a moderately increased blood pressure (average 164/89 mm of Hg) can adversely affect performance on cognitive tests. Obviously, such microscopic changes in brain can result in overt problems. These are observed through progressive increase in sensory problems such as visual and hearing loss; these problems are compounded by an increase in their respective signal-to-noise ratio. Other problems involve decline in word retrieval and memory, which is demonstrated through lower scores and longer response times on cognitive tests. Also compromised are motor movements relating to balance and equilibrium, as well as coordination of fine motor acts.

Recent literature however, fosters optimism through reports of some positive findings in the aging nervous system. Studies of animal models have confirmed the presence of neurogenesis in hippocampus; the addition of new neurons in this region is perhaps related to its significance for establishing new memories and learning. Also, there is increasing evidence supporting the concept of "use it or lose it;" it has been proven that new and mature neurons thrive in positive, active and stimulating environment. For example, participating in regular physical activity has shown to improve metabolic performance and is associated with longevity. Finally, it is speculated that age-related differences in memory are related to storage capacity, and not to processing efficiency. This contention is promising since it implies that we maintain the ability to learn and recall information even if we run out of places to store new information.

SUMMARY

The brain has the unique ability to serve as a multitask, multiprocessing organ. This capability enables it to perform routine bodily functions and at the same time attend to its self-growth. An understanding of its functional organization alerts one to assess its myriad functions, and their influence on each other, in the event of brain damage. Like any other organ, the brain, too, undergoes changes with age progression; some of these alterations have negative implications, but there is some reassuring information as well. At this stage it is unclear if anatomical changes in neural tissue lead to physiological aging, or if these two factors are mutually exclusive.

Chapter 5

ETIOLOGIES AND
NEURODIAGNOSTIC TESTS

The most common cause for communication problems in adults is stroke, or *cerebrovascular accident (CVA),* which is defined as the disruption of the blood flow to the brain resulting in deprivation of oxygen to the cerebral tissue. The disruption may be sudden or slow, and it may result from several possible etiologies and medical diagnoses. The contemporary term "brain attack" is used to stress the similarities between a CVA and heart attack, and emphasize the fact that each of these conditions is preventable and treatable in victims of strokes.

The signs and symptoms of a CVA may be presented as a combination of one or more of the following reports: sudden unexplained dizziness or clumsiness; numbness of face, arm, leg, or one side of the body; loss of consciousness; cramps after exercise; undue flushing of the face; inability to speak or trouble talking or understanding speech; sudden dimming or loss of vision, especially in one eye; sudden severe headache with no known cause; vomiting; and paresis (weakness) or paralysis of an arm or leg or both.

While strokes can be deadly, the majority of people who have a stroke survive with mild to severe persisting disability. Of the 2.5 million persons who suffer from CVA at a given time, approximately 20–21 percent will have some communication problem. The primary etiologies for neurogenic communication disorders are distributed as follows: CVA (64%), traumatic brain injury (TBI; 25%), and other neurological conditions (11%). This Chapter therefore, describes the different etiologic (causative) groups with related risk and background factors (see Table 5.1). It also reviews some of the pertinent neurodiagnostic tests that help determine the type, location and extent of the brain damage.

RISK FACTORS

Every minute someone in the United States experiences a stroke; therefore, it has been considered the leading cause of adult disability, and the third leading cause of death in the Country. Nearly everyone has the potential to have a stroke, however, there is adequate demographic evidence to show that the incidence of CVA is influenced by several risk factors including age, gender, ethnicity, and pre-existing medical conditions. Overall, the risk of having a stroke doubles with each decade past age 55. The likelihood of getting a CVA is one in 1,000 for individuals who are in the 50-year age group; this number increases to 10 per 1,000 among those in their 70s, and doubles to 20 per 1,000 in the age 80 group. Men are at a higher risk than females for having a stroke; however, because women in the United States live longer than men, most stroke survivors over age 65 are women. African Americans are almost twice as likely to have a CVA and die from it as white Americans.

Pre-existing conditions such as diabetes, previous CVA, and family history increase the probability of acquiring a CVA. Individuals with diabetes, or high blood sugar, have a higher risk of stroke perhaps due to the impaired glucose metabolism caused by the disease. Also, the risk of a second CVA multiplies 10 times for people who have had an earlier attack. Finally, a family history of stroke predisposes an individual to acquire a CVA as well. The welcoming news is that medical advances in diagnostic procedures and management have made a positive impact on reducing the incidence, severity, and mortality rates from strokes. For example, if the CVA results from a blood clot or blocked arteries, many times medication and/or surgery can reduce the severity of its effect and also lower the possibility of having another one.

Risk factors for stroke are similar to those for cardiovascular disease because both conditions are related to arteriosclerosis. Heart disease due to atrial fibrillation, high blood pressure and heart valve inadequacy can increase the risk of stroke. *Atrial fibrillation* causes the upper left chamber of the heart to beat erratically and unpredictably; it increases the risk for stroke by allowing blood to pool in the heart and form clots that can then be carried to the brain. Similarly, heart valve problems can lead to clot formation and consequently impede blood flow to the brain. High blood pressure, or *hypertension,* is a risk factor that often can be controlled with proper exercise, a low-salt/low-fat diet, anticoagulant medication, smoking cessation and weight loss (Hacke, Hennerici, Gelmers & Krämer, 1991). Other risk factors relate to lifestyle, and one of them is smoking. Smoking damages the arterial walls, speeds up the clogging of arteries, raises blood pressure, and makes the heart work harder. High levels of blood cholesterol, being overweight, leading a sedentary lifestyle, and excessive alcohol consumption are also associated with increased stroke risk.

ISCHEMIC CVA: OCCLUSIVE TYPES

According to the *World Health Organization* and the *American Heart Association,* the majority (approximately 80%) of all stroke victims have an ischemic CVA. *Ischemia* is a condition when cerebral blood flow falls below the required level for normal cell metabolism and function. It is therefore, associated with vascular disturbances that result in either total *occlusion* (obstruction) or partial constriction (*stenosis*) of a blood vessel. Some examples of occlusive ischemic CVAs are thrombosis, embolism and arteriosclerosis (see Table 5.1 and Figure 5.1); each of these conditions are described in this section.

Thrombosis, or *thrombotic CVA,* accounts for two-thirds of all ischemic CVAs in individuals over 60 years. This diagnosis implies an obstruction of a blood vessel generally caused by a *thrombus* which is a blood clot or a plug in the vessel remaining at the point of its formation. The thrombus prevents the artery from supplying blood to its distribution area thus resulting in thrombosis. Thrombosis may occur secondary to a cardiac disease, diabetes, endarteritis, arteriosclerosis, syphilis, or trauma.

Embolism (or *Embolic CVA*) can occur in any age group, and accounts for nearly ten percent of all CVAs. This condition also results from total obstruction of a blood vessel, however, the inflicted artery is generally smaller in diameter than that affected in thrombosis. The obstructive agent, an *embolus,* can be a small substance in the form of a blood clot, plaque or other body tissue that may travel from remote

Table 5.1. Major Etiologies and Diagnoses for Neurogenic Communication Disorders.

Ischemic CVA	Traumatic Brain Injury	Infections	Degenerative Diseases	Other Conditions
Thrombosis	Open head injury	Meningitis	Multi-infarct CVA	Brain tumor
Embolism	Closed head injury	Encephalitis	Pick's disease	Normal pressure hydrocephalus
Arteriosclerosis	Diffuse axonal injury	Cerebral abscess	Alzheimer's disease	Epilepsy
Aneurysm		Rheumatic disease	Creuzfeldt-Jacob disease	Substance abuse
Cerebral hemorrhage		Leukemia	Progressive supranuclear palsy	Neurotoxin exposure
Arterio-venous malformation		Sickle cell disease	Parkinson's disease	Anoxia
Transient ischemic attack			Huntington's disease	Posttraumatic syndrome

areas of the body until it plugs up a vessel that is smaller than its size. Therefore, embolism is not necessarily local in its origin and effect. Embolism has been associated with pre-existing conditions such as cardiac problems, arteriosclerosis, or pulmonary disorders.

Both thrombosis and embolism can result in deprivation of blood flow to the brain, or *cerebral infarction.* An *infarct* is a focal deadened area, while infarction is the process that leads to death or destruction of the cerebral tissue.

Arteriosclerosis accounts for 60 percent of all ischemic CVAs. Because this condition is insidious, it calls for a brief review of the progressive changes in the arterial structure and function. Normally, an artery has three layers of tissue, two of which are elastic to allow it to expand and constrict to circulate the blood. Any damage to the arterial wall is repaired by deposition of *plaque,* a whitish substance that is formed with the help of blood cholesterol and other materials such as calcium. The key component of cholesterol is nonmetabolized low density lipoprotein (or LDL). Plaque formation results from accumulation of LDL, which attracts scavenging white blood cells (monocytes) to stick to arterial walls and engulf the cholesterol passing in the bloodstream. The white cells typically start burrowing between layers of arterial wall, damaging it in the process as well. The accumulation of LDL results in oxidation (analogous to rusting of pipes) and glycation (binding by sugars). In time, the build-up of plaque can calcify and solidify to lessen the elasticity of the arterial walls, which is commonly described as "hardening" of the arteries and marks the beginning of arteriosclerosis. Progressively, plaque hangings from the wall lead to constriction of the lumen of the arteries, or *stenosis,* and impede the blood flow to the target sites. The slowing down of blood flow increases the risk of clot formation and the possibility of a thrombosis; or a piece of plaque may get dislodged to form an embolus and travel with the blood to block a smaller, remote vessel and result in an embolism.

Some risk factors for arteriosclerosis are high fat content in diet, which increases blood cholesterol (LDL) levels. Obesity contributes to diabetes, which can elevate glucose levels in blood and enhance glycation, which in turn, may hasten the oxidation of LDL. Another factor includes smoking, which causes formation of oxidants and foster oxidation as well. Finally, hypertension increases the vulnerability of the arterial walls to inflammation and consequently to plaque formation (Libby, 2002).

There is some distinction between arteriosclerosis and *atherosclerosis* (or *atheroma*). Atherosclerosis implies degeneration of arterial walls associated with the aging process. It generally begins in large vessels where plaque deposits are concentrated at locations where the arteries branch or bend sharply. The alteration in the force of blood flow on artery walls at such vulnerable locations perhaps triggers the onset of plaque formation. For example, plaque may first be found at the branching of common carotid artery just beyond its bulbous swelling, or in the intra-osseous portion of the vertebral and basilar arteries.

Transient Ischemic Attacks (TIA), also known as the "Syndrome of Intermittent Insufficiency of the Internal Carotid System," represent warning signs of an underlying vascular problem in the brain. The symptoms of TIA mimic some of the CVA symptoms, however, the symptoms may diminish relatively quickly within a few minutes to a few hours; unlike CVA, TIA does not result in permanent disability. Having a TIA can increase an individual's risk for a stroke by 10 times; approximately one of three patients with TIA develop a CVA within five years. The underlying cause of TIA is related to stenotic arteries and possibly caused by arteriosclerosis, hypertension (fluctuating type), anemia, or thyroid disorders. Treating the first episode of TIA can greatly reduce the risk of incurring a CVA.

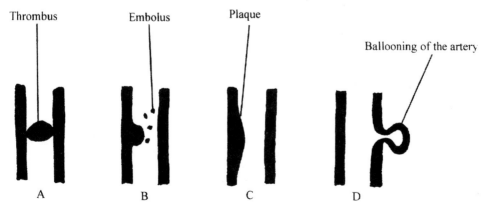

Figure 5.1. Ischemic cerebrovascular accidents resulting from thrombosis (A), embolism (B), arteriosclerosis (C), and aneurysm (D).

ISCHEMIC CVA: NONOCCLUSIVE TYPES

A nonocclusive ischemic CVA is the consequence of a vascular problem, but there is no obstruction of the affected blood vessel. Some examples of nonocclusive ischemic CVAs include aneurysm, cerebral hemorrhage and arteriovenous malformation:

Aneurysm is a structural abnormality of a blood vessel, which originated from a congenital weakness during the formation of arterial walls. It may remain undiagnosed until adulthood, and may be detected only when the weakened area has progressively stretched and ballooned out as a sac. If the aneurysm is present in one of the arteries supplying the brain, then the individual may manifest symptoms of TIA, which if ignored, may lead to rupture of the aneurysm and consequently to a cerebral hemorrhage (see Figure 5.1).

Cerebral hemorrhage, or *hemorrhagic CVA,* occurs when an artery to the brain bursts or bleeds. This type of stroke accounts for 30 percent of all CVAs and it is more often fatal than an occlusive CVA. The bleeding in the brain may result from a head trauma, excessive hypertension, or a ruptured aneurysm. A hemorrhage that has congealed to form a clot, or *hematoma,* is sometimes considered the lesser of the two evils. Two major categories of cerebral hemorrhages or hematoma have been described (see Figure 5.2): intracranial, and intracerebral. An *intracranial hemorrhage* (or hematoma) is determined if the bleeding (or clot) occurs within the skull and the meninges. If it occurs in the epidural space (between the duramater and the skull), then an *epidural hemorrhage* (or hematoma) is determined; correspondingly, a *subdural hemorrhage* (bleeding between the dura and arachnoid mater), or a subarachnoid hemorrhage (bleeding between the arachnoid and pia mater) is also possible. In contrast, *intracerebral hemorrhage* implies that there is bleeding directly on the cerebral tissue and therefore, it has the most severe consequences. The presence of any of these types of hemorrhages (or hematoma) can compress the brain tissue thus increasing *intracranial pressure.*

Arterio-Venous Malformation (AVM) is also an indicator of a congenital problem because it reflects the failure of embryonic blood vessels to mature and establish themselves as either arteries or veins; thus the blood vessels in the AVM are not clearly distinguishable in their functions as either arteries or veins. This structural flaw creates a mixing of oxygenated and deoxygenated blood in the affected area, which may disrupt brain function resulting in the symptoms of a TIA or CVA.

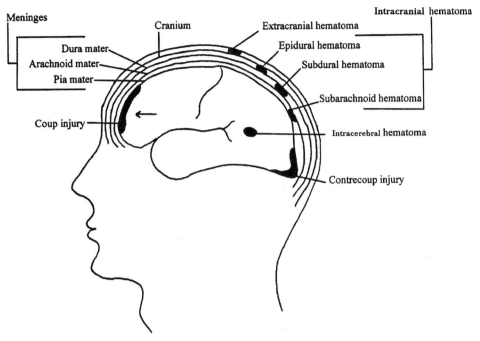

Figure 5.2. Types of head injuries and possible locations for hematomas (or hemorrhages).

HEAD INJURY

Also known as *Traumatic Brain Injury* (TBI), it is a lesion to the brain due to sudden head acceleration followed by an abrupt deceleration; it is broadly identified as either an *open* or *closed head injury* dependent upon the integrity of the skull and superficial tissue. TBI is one of the leading causes for brain damage and it is the number one killer of persons under age 34; the majority of its victims are between 15 and 24 years (Adamovich, 1998). Each year approximately a million brain injuries occur in the United States; of these, approximately 373,000 require hospitalization and an estimated 56,000 people die each year. Motor vehicle accident is the primary cause of TBI (50%), followed by falls (21%), firearms (12%), and sport and recreation (10%) injuries. Nearly one-third of persons with TBI need some form of speech-language therapy.

Effects of a head injury may range from concussion to coma. A *concussion* is severe jarring of the cerebral tissue with no visible signs of a trauma; in such instance, the victim may report experiencing headache, nausea, dizziness, or concentration problems. A *contusion* is a visible bruise from the injury, but the skin is not torn. In severe cases the individual may go in a *coma,* which is a period of unconsciousness and unresponsiveness. A coma may last from hours to weeks; the length of coma has been accepted as a prognostic indicator for the recovery from the head injury. Sometimes the individual may be in a *vegetative state* when the cardiovascular and respiration may be functioning, the eyes may be open, but the patient does not respond or communicate. Other symptoms associated with acute TBI may include seizures, bradycardia and widened pulse pressure, intracranial hemorrhage, head and neck stiffness, visual problems (retinal hemorrhage, diplopia, pupil dilation, inability to track objects), hearing problems (CSF or blood leakage in ear, unilateral hearing loss) and vomiting due to increased intracranial pressure.

The concept of *diffuse axonal injury* is associated with nonimpact jarring of the brain from a TBI or any form of speed-related activity as in players colliding while engaged in contact sports such as football. The shearing forces in the brain from abrupt changes in velocity are enough to cause microscopic damage to the nerve fibers. Minor blows to the head once regarded inconsequential can also produce long-term effects. The damage is not visible during routine laboratory tests, but it can cause short and long-term symptoms including dizziness, headache, fatigue, irritability, as well as attention and memory disturbances. Diffuse axonal injury can also launch an insidiously progressive neurodegenerative process, which can take years to unfold and develop/mimic plaque-forming process and mild cognitive impairments associated with symptoms of Alzheimer's disease.

CEREBRAL INFLAMMATION

A variety of bacterial or viral infection, or inflammation, may also cause brain damage (see Table 5.1). The brain's reaction to the foreign invasion may be acute (or immediate) or it may be chronic (long-lasting). Common examples of acute infection in the brain are meningitis and encephalitis. *Meningitis* is inflammation of the meninges; the bacterial or viral organism invade the blood stream, constrict the lumen of the arteries, increase intracranial pressure, and ultimately damages the neural tissue. The inflammatory reaction may be relatively severe in case of bacterial meningitis than for the viral form. *Encephalitis* is a generalized viral infection of the cerebral tissue, which may also lead to abscess formation and brain damage as well. Possible complications of acute meningitis or encephalitis are seizures, coma, and even death. A *cerebral abscess* is a defined as local destruction of tissue resulting from either an acute or a chronic infection of the brain.

Chronic long-term diseases such as *rheumatic disease, syphilis, leukemia,* or *sickle cell disease* can also cause brain damage. In each of these conditions the vascular system is compromised and therefore, there may be disruption of blood flow to the brain. For example, the heart valve may be impaired as a complication of rheumatic (fever) disease; the arterial walls may be damaged in syphilis and leukemia; and the deformed red blood cells in sickle cell disease may increase blood viscosity and lead to clot formation and occlusive CVA.

NEURODEGENERATIVE DISEASES

The term *neurodegeneration* implies a gradual wasting of neural tissue. The course of degeneration may be *progressive* (or *irreversible*) implying that it cannot be arrested. The degeneration may begin at the cortical (cerebral cortex) level, or at the subcortical (corpus striatum or brainstem) level; occasionally, it is referred as mixed if it involves both cortical and subcortical structures. This section describes some degenerative diseases that generally show the onset of dementia as its early and primary problem (see Table 5.1).

Multi-infarct CVA involves the presence or history of several episodes of vascular lesions resulting in multiple areas of infarctions and as such it presents a combination of mixed, cortical and subcortical clinical features. Approximately 10–15 percent of dementias are attributed to multi-infarct CVAs, which are generally associated with advanced atherosclerotic changes in one or more of the arteries of the brain.

Pick's disease is a rare disorder that is considered "presenile dementia" because it generally affects relatively younger adults usually between ages 40–60, but it has been found to range from 20–80 years. Pick's disease is characterized by slow, progressive deterioration of frontal or temporal lobes or both, and tends to be familial in nature.

Alzheimer's disease (AD) is named after the German neurologist who first described his patient's symptoms in 1906. This disease has perhaps received the most attention because it contributes to two-thirds of all dementias, and it is also referred as dementia of the *Alzheimer's type* (DAT). The incidence of AD is 2–4 million of the population and it is associated with advancing age. About 100,000 persons die from AD each year, and it is deemed the fourth leading cause of death in the United States.

If AD occurs before age 60, or between 30–45 years, then it is classified as *early onset*/presenile dementia/*familial AD;* its suspected cause is defective chromosome 14.

Late onset AD is considered senile dementia since the symptoms begin after age 60. This variant of AD is associated with mutation on chromosome 12 (C12) and some report mutation of chromosome 21 (C21), which is also associated with Down's syndrome. Mutation of C21 results in reduced acetylcholine production, which affects production of "amyloid precursor protein" (APP); this event results in beta amyloid deposits, which although found throughout the body in harmless form, can change and form toxic strands that build up on brain cells. The amyloid production leads to formation of neurofibrillary tangles inside the neurons and neuritic plaques outside the neurons. Such formations are seen in high concentration in the hippocampus, septum pellucidum and in the neocortex. There are also high levels of a gene apoliproprotein-E4 (or ApoE) in AD; this occurrence is also associated with greater demyelination of white matter in AD. If a person has high levels of ApoE, and a history of head injury, then this individual is ten times likely to develop DAT. Finally, higher concentration of aluminum (50 times greater than normal), which destroys the neurons, has also been found in individuals with AD.

Nongenetic factors have also been associated with AD. For example, study of twins shows that both twins do not get AD; also, there is a higher incidence of DAT in children born to younger fathers. Another risk factor is poor linguistic ability in early life as determined from the longitudinal study of 93 nuns; this association was verified through analyses of 25 brains at autopsy and corresponding linguistic quality of one-page written biographical samples from the nuns when they were in their 20s.

Other degenerative diseases that also manifest symptoms of dementia include *Creutzfeldt-Jakob disease* and progressive supranuclear palsy. Creutzfeldt-Jakob disease (CJD) is a rare (one per million), idiopathic form of progressive disease where rogue proteins, or *prions,* gradually destroy the neural tissue. Normally, this incurable disease is seen in people 45 years and older; however, it is possible to acquire a variant form of CJD from consumption of meat infected with bovine spongiform encephalopathy (BSE) at any age. The variant form of CJD has been identified since the early 1990s in both Europe and North America. *Progressive supranuclear palsy* is a bilateral subcortical degeneration which gradually progresses to involve the cortical tissue and result in dementia during the advanced stages of the disease.

OTHER CONDITIONS

This category includes a collection of conditions that may also disrupt normal brain functions (see Table 5.1). Some examples of these disorders include brain tumor, epilepsy, substance abuse, and anoxia as probable causes of acquired brain damage.

Brain Tumors are sometimes described as space occupying lesions since they tend to infiltrate, crowd out the healthy neural tissue, and increase the intracranial CSF pressure. Tumors in the brain develop from neuroglia, typically from astrocytes or oligodendrocytes and thus diagnosed as *astrocytoma* or *oligodendroglioma* or *glioma.* The severity of the tumor is determined based on the degree of its malignancy (low grade versus high grade) and its location in the brain. Low grade (grade I) tumors tend to be slow growing and are sometimes considered as "benign" tumors. At the opposite end of the spectrum are aggressive, fast growing tumors such as the *glioblastoma multiform.* The location of the tumor is of equal consideration. For example, a tumor in the central core of the brain deep within the diencephalon or within the brainstem structures is life-threatening because of the difficulty in reaching the tumor without damaging adjacent structures that are critical for survival.

Occasionally, the presence of *pseudotumor cerebri* may create a diagnostic confusion between true brain tumor, meningitis, or cerebral hemorrhage because the symptoms in each of these conditions tend to be similar. Unlike the other three conditions, pseudotumor cerebri results from imbalanced production and absorption of CSF perhaps related to hormonal imbalance in females between 20–40 years. A recent label, *normal pressure hydrocephalus* (NPH), is used to refer to disrupted CSF flow among older adults. In the majority of cases, NPH is idiopathic in origin, however, in some individuals NPH is associated with predisposing conditions such as TBI, brain tumor or cysts, hematoma or hemorrhage, or inflammation. The CSF is impeded in its flow within the brain resulting in its accumulation in the ventricles and increased CSF pressure. The triad of symptoms in older adults with NPH includes gait disturbance, mild dementia and impaired bladder control (Hydrocephalus Association, 2002).

Epilepsy, or idiopathic seizures, is electrical storms in either local or large areas of the brain, which are manifested as abnormal muscular activity (or seizures). *Rasmussen's encephalopathy,* an autoimmune disorder, is an example of idiopathic progressive increase in seizures in young children. The seizures begin as mild, focal muscle tremors and increase to 100 plus full-blown muscle spasms per day. Nonidiopathic (or symptomatic) seizures can occur as a consequence of an ischemic CVA, head trauma, or brain tumor. The intensity and duration of seizure activity may vary; if they are fleeting in occurrence and involve a small group of local muscles as in muscle twitch or tremor, then they are referred as *petit mal* seizures. Whenever large number of muscles indulges into a collective spasm, then it is termed *grand mal* seizures. A third type, *Jacksonian* seizures refer to a progression of spasms from a local group of muscles, which serve as trigger points, until the convulsions spread to other muscles and engulf the entire body.

Substance abuse, or use of recreational drugs in the form of continual use of stimulants or depressants can also lead to brain damage. Drug addiction is considered a learned behavior resulting from the strengthening of connections between the brain's reward circuits and learning and memory. Both stimulants and depressants tend to block off, or adversely affect the release and re-uptake of neurotransmitters. Chronic drug use can directly produce permanent brain dysfunction, or it can first affect the vascular system which in turn can lead to an ischemic CVA. Examples of stimulants include amphetamine compounds (methamphetamines or "speed"), cocaine (and its higher dose "crack"), steroids, solvents, nitrites, and antidepressants. A common effect of such drugs is elevated blood pressure, heart rate and blood velocity, which can increase the risk for a CVA particularly if taken by individuals with a history of hypertension or a vulnerable cardiovascular system. Phenylpropanolamine (PPA) is chemically similar to methamphetamine and is marketed alone or in combination with other agents and is found in almost 70 over-the-counter products such as diet aids (appetite suppressants), cold medications, decongestants, antihistamines, caffeine, vitamins, benzocaine and fructose. Methamphetamine is more potent than cocaine because it tends to remain in the brain longer and is not flushed out as quickly as cocaine. Its overdose or abuse results in hypertension, respiratory problems and ischemic CVAs (hemorrhagic, thrombotic) due to constriction and inflammation of blood vessels. Methamphetamine greatly damages the cells in the limbic system particularly the hippocampus and the cingulum, which are also affected by the early stages of Alzheimer's disease. The adverse effects of such stimulant drugs is manifested as increased agitation, anxiety, psychosis, confusion and disorientation, perceptual disorders, memory disturbance, and attention problems.

Depressants, or calmative drugs sedate cortical activity by stimulating lower, subcortical levels; they tend to influence serotonin activity in the brain. Some examples of these drugs are angel dust (phencyclidine or PCP/"angel dust"), opium (e.g., fentanyl), sedatives, and hallucinogens (e.g., LSD). Opiates in the form of heroin, morphine and meperidines (Demerol) mimic the brain's natural opioids (endorphins and encephalins) to produce temporary euphoria; their repeated use can deplete the brain's neurotransmitters. Sedatives such as barbiturates (phenobarbitol/Luminol) and benzodiazepines (valium, Halcion, Xanax) reduce excitatory synaptic activity by facilitating the release of inhibitory transmitters (Templer, Hartlage & Cannon, 1992).

Alcohol consumption as a form of substance abuse is frequently associated with TBI; 40–66 percent of TBI victims have a history of pre-injury alcohol abuse and 27–50 percent of these individuals have post-injury abuse. Alcohol combined with other recreational drugs is a lethal combination for potential brain damage. Continuation of these habits can also interfere with rehabilitation and recovery as reflected through poor compliancy, increased depression, and increased risk for additional injury (falls) and other health complications.

Neurotoxins are environmental or industrial compounds that can have an adverse effect on brain function as well. One group of neurotoxins includes compounds that have metals such as arsenic, lead, manganese, mercury and tin (or organtin). Another equally dangerous group of toxins are organic solvents that can extract, dissolve, or suspend nonwater soluble materials such as fats, oils, resins, waxes, plastics, polymers, and cellulose derivatives. These compounds can be found in household and agricultural products, and thus it is not surprising that they can increase the risk for brain damage.

Anoxia, or oxygen deprivation to the brain from vascular insufficiency may result from cardiac problems such as coronary thrombosis (heart attack) or myocardial infarction (cardiac insufficiency). Anoxia can result in degeneration of neurons with the cellular destruction proceeding in the following order:

- At normal body temperature, five minutes of circulatory/cardiac arrest depletes the glucose reserve in the brain and marks the onset of brain damage.
- In 10 minutes the brain uses up its oxygen reserve; this event causes the neurons to release glutamate, which binds with nearby receptors to allow rapid influx of elements such as calcium into the cell. To compensate for the toxic levels of calcium the cells draw in more water, which leads to swelling and eventual bursting of the neuron. In brief, glutamate is the culprit that kills the neurons and leads to necrosis (death) and liquidation of the brain.
- Within 24 hours degenerative changes in neurons are seen through *chromatolysis,* which characterizes displacement of the nucleus and disappearance of soma.
- In a few days the brain tissue disintegrates completely and is replaced by a large number of spherical, scavenger cells with abundant cytoplasm; this is the first visible sign of infarction. The term *brain death* implies the irreversible cessation of function of brain structures, including the cerebellum and brainstem structures.

Two other factors, microwave radiation and nerve gas exposure, have also been identified as potential causatives for brain damage. *Microwave radiation* emitted from mobile phones has been linked to brain damage in rats exposed to minimum two hours of continuous exposure for over a one-month period. There is some evidence of brain damage among soldiers suffering from *posttraumatic (war) syndrome.* Some of the speculated causes for the disrupted brain function may have been the result of combined effects of exposure to prolonged stress, low-level nerve gas exposure and antigas tablets taken by the soldiers during the recent gulf war. Some examples of cognitive impairments associated with Gulf-war syndrome include confusion, memory lapses and depression.

TESTS FOR MEDICAL DIAGNOSIS
AND LESION LOCALIZATION

Medical verification of overt symptoms is made through the collection of information from at least one or more laboratory test results. Select tests are prescribed for individuals at risk or with suspected brain damage; they aim to provide anatomical information regarding the size and location of lesion, as well as the physiological status of the damaged and adjacent nondamaged areas. The results from such neurodiagnostic tests help verify the medical diagnosis and make decisions regarding further assessment, referral and intervention. Some of the related procedures are therefore described in this section.

Computerized Axial Tomography (CAT/CT scan) was introduced for clinical use during the 1970s. The CT scanning procedure involves exposure to a series of x-rays beamed at 2–10 mm intervals swiveling in a full circle around the head. Each of these sets of beams absorbed by the different structures and represented as a transverse section of brain. Series of such consecutive sections, displaying density (bone versus other tissue) differences, help visualize the size and site of the infarcted area. This procedure is required prior to administering any form of anticoagulants (or blood thinners) to patients with occlusive CVAs in order to rule out any active hemorrhaging in the brain. It is cautioned that a CT scan may not yield details regarding the size and location of the damage if the test is performed immediately after the onset of a CVA.

Magnetic Resonance Imaging (MRI), evolved from *Nuclear Magnetic Resonance* (NMR) of the 1950s, found its clinical niche in the 1980s. This procedure entails exposure to a magnetic field of 3000 gauss (or 1.5 tesla), which excites the hydrogen atoms and other odd number of protons and neutrons in the body to orient with the instrument's magnetic field just like a compass needle. When the magnet is turned off the spinning (resonating) atoms release energy in the form of radio waves called "Larmor" frequency, which provides a measure of hydrogen concentration in different tissue types. The resulting image displays different tissue densities thus differentiating gray versus white matter, CSF flow and any pathological anomaly. The MRI images can be stacked to form a three-dimensional model of the brain that can be re-sliced along any plane or angle.

Although both MRI and CT scans provide anatomical information, the MRI has some advantages over the CT scan. The MRI does not involve exposure to radiation; it permits unlimited viewing angles and slices and planes (sagittal, horizontal, coronal), and the image depiction is not constrained by bone. The MRI procedure also encounters some obstacles. For example, individuals wearing pacemakers or metal implants may not be candidates, nor may people with claustrophobic reactions. Also, the image collection time for MRI is longer than for CT scan and therefore, it is a lengthier procedure.

Some derivations of the standard MRI procedure have also been introduced in recent years. Such modifications focus on evaluating brain function and they are considered as *brain mapping* applications of MRI. Examples include the following options:

- *MR Spectroscopy* analyzes chemical composition of body tissue including the brain. For example, it can detect abnormal growth without needing biopsy, or provide the chemical profile of an organ, or determine the effect of medication on the target organ.
- *MR Projection Angiography* helps view the blood vessels, as well as assess the blood flow in target arteries. This application is useful for the diagnosis of occlusive ischemic CVAs.
- *Magnetoencephalography* (MEG) is based on the contention that the flow of sodium and potassium ions produces a magnetic field which, although weak, is detectable by the recording device is called SQUID (Superconducting Quantum Interference Device). This procedure helps observe neural activity and differentiate normal from abnormal processing of brain signals. The MEG has been used in individuals with epilepsy, CVA, Alzheimer's disease, coma, spinal cord injury, migraines, narcolepsy, and learning disability.
- *Functional Magnetic Resonance Imaging* (fMRI) technique detects blood-oxygen level in select areas of the brain. For example, when an area is functionally active, capillaries respond to its need for increased blood flow by dilating and allowing more oxygen to enter the area. The fMRI is capable of observing microscopic changes in blood flow to differentiate active versus resting (or damaged) areas; thus it can track the normal and pathological functions of the brain from pre-op through recovery in individuals who are candidates for AVM or tumor extraction surgeries.
- *MRI–Tensor Diffusion Imaging* utilizes a special software to measure the direction and speed of water as it flows/diffuses in the nerve

fibers. This information helps diagnose the amount of nerve damage in individuals with multiple sclerosis.

Spinal Tap/Lumbar Puncture involves an analysis of the CSF to detect internal bleeding (may appear pink or bloody), possible infection and immunological status, and CSF pressure to confirm pseudotumor cerebri. The procedure is performed under local anesthesia to withdraw CSF from the lower back, between the second and third lumbar vertebrae. Some adverse effects of spinal tap may include the possibility of developing meningitis, headache, vomiting, neck stiffness, and cartilage rupture.

Electroencephalography (EEG) involves the use of 22–32 surface electrodes, which are symmetrically placed on identical locations on both sides of the brain using the standard "10–20 system." The electrodes record the degree and symmetry of surface brain activity from the different locations. The obtained EEG tracings are evaluated as either normal or abnormal; for example, there may be increased activity during seizures, or decreased activity in an infarcted area.

A popular outgrowth of EEG is *Evoked* (or *Event Related*) *Potentials,* which records brain's responses to visual (VER), auditory (AER or ABR), or proprioceptive stimulation. The evoked potentials detect possible dysfunction in the transmission of signals between the corresponding cranial (sensory) nerves and the brainstem; they also provide information regarding brain's attention to each of these stimuli. Another application, the *Brain Electrical Activity Mapping* (BEAM) utilizes computer programs to display evoked potentials as lateral view images of the brain; the stimulated areas are generally depicted as enhanced/illuminated areas. The BEAM has been used in research on Alzheimer's disease, learning disability, and psychiatric disorders.

Brain Scan (*Cerebral Scintigraphy/Isotope Scanning/Radionucleide Scanning*) utilizes radioactive (isotope) material, which is injected in the carotid artery via a catheter inserted in the femoral artery. Series of x-rays, or videotaped images are taken as the isotope travels in blood to the brain. The infarcted areas absorb the isotope and are thus identified in the visual images to circumscribe the size and location of cerebral damage.

Cerebral Arteriography or *Angiography* involves the injection of a radio opaque dye, which is less powerful than an isotope, into the carotid or vertebral artery via a catheter inserted in the femoral artery. Similar to brain scanning, the circulating dye helps examine the diameter of arteries, degree of stenosis, location of the occlusion, presence of single versus multiple occlusions, and existence and state of collateral circulation. A derivative of this procedure, *digitized intravenous arteriography,* is performed in patients who are too ill to undergo routine arteriography. The radio opaque dye is injected in the vein, and it is diluted by the time it reaches brain (vein → lung → heart → artery → brain) thus minimizing possible complications or side effects from the dye.

Doppler sonography (*Ultrasonography/Ultrasound imaging/Echoencephalography*) entails the use of high frequency sound waves, between 3 and 7 MHz (30,000–70,000 Hz), which are transmitted by a transducer held against the target region. Echoes of these sound waves bounce back; they are detected by the same transducer and displayed as visual images. Degree of absorption and scattering of sound waves vary with body tissue; these differences in the returning echoes reveal structural features of the neural tissue. The primary limitation of doppler sonography is that it does not provide as wide a field of view as the MRI. Some of its applications include the following procedures:

- *Invasive Ultrasound* is used during neurosurgery to guide the surgeon around sensitive areas or blood vessels; it also helps identify tumors and abscesses that are difficult to detect by eye and helps assure that excessive tissue is not removed.
- *Ultrasound catheter* (*and imaging*) is used to examine the degree of stenosis of the internal carotid or any other artery. The computer detects any change in the sound/tone to form the visual image (or *sonic snapshot*) of the artery.
- *Brain injury scanner* is a helmet-like device with two transducers at the temples that send low frequency ultrasound signals through the brain to determine the presence of bleeding, blood clot or other anomaly.

Positron Emission Tomography (PET) scan displays the metabolic status or changes that reflect brain function. The patient either inhales or receives an intravenous injection of "positron emitters" (metabolically important substances such as carbon, oxygen, nitrogen, glucose or ammonia) combined with "tracers" (mildly radioactive isotope such as Xenon 133). The isotope concentrates in areas that consume the positron emitters; the reaction between the positron emitters and the neighboring electrons give rise to gamma rays (radiation), which are detected by the computer to generate visual images. Active, absorbing areas light up while those that do not absorb the emitters remain as darker areas. The isotope dissolves and returns to harmless state within 15–30 minutes. PET scans have been used in several applications: assess blood flow after a CVA; examine individuals with epilepsy, Alzheimer's disease, or tumors; evaluate the effect of medications in Parkinson's or Huntington's disease; and observe anxiety effects when anticipating pain/shock and in panic disorders. A derivative, *Single Photon Emission Computed Tomography* (SPECT), is more cost-effective and readily available. It utilizes only those isotopes approved by the *Food and Drug Administration* (FDA) and allows measurement of *Regional Cerebral Blood Flow* (rCBF), which entails inhaling Xenon 133.

SUMMARY

Brain performance is dependent on optimal supply of oxygen, glucose and related nutrients and electrolytes that are delivered at precise blood pressure. When the supply of these metabolic requirements is disrupted, the brain reacts by manifesting a collection of dysfunctions that are overtly observed as clinical symptoms. It is these symptoms that initiate a volley of diagnostic tests with the aim to determine the precise cause of the disrupted cerebral function and lead to a medical diagnosis. Information from the medical diagnostic procedures also establishes an understanding of the size and location of the cerebral lesion. Selection of an appropriate assessment protocol is vital to ascertain the diagnosis and formulate a plan for management or alleviation of the causative condition. Each of these preceding steps is also vital for understanding the nature of the communication disorder and determining possible prognosis and intervention options for the residual symptoms.

Chapter 6

COMMUNICATION DISORDERS
AND RELATED SYMPTOMS

The consequences of brain damage are myriad. Of the different possible symptoms, those contributing directly or indirectly to disrupted human communication are described in this chapter. Normal communicative interactions result from an integration of linguistic, sensory-perceptual, cognitive and motor functions. The goal of this chapter is to define each of these groups of symptoms and to direct attention to their interrelationships, as well as diagnostic labels such as aphasia and cognitive-communication disorders associated with traumatic brain injury, right hemisphere lesions, and dementia. Of equal consideration is developing an understanding that the different symptoms are related to the underlying location/site of lesion, which may involve either the right or left hemisphere, or the cortical or subcortical structures.

APHASIA

The term *aphasia,* also known as *dysphasia,* was first introduced in 1864 by Trousseau to imply loss of speech and writing. Aphasia simply refers to disordered language that is generally associated with lesions involving the language-dominant (left) hemisphere. This concise definition, however, has undergone a gradual evolution since its introduction. During the 1940s–1950s, the definition of aphasia was elaborated to include the possibility of either "receptive" (or comprehension/decoding) or "expressive" (or production/encoding) language disorder. This dichotomy was reflected in the definitions proposed by some prominent authorities of this period. For example, Henry Head defined aphasia as an impairment of symbolic formulation and expression; and Berry and Eisenson described it as the disturbance in the ability to comprehend visual or auditory communicative symbols, or to produce words, phrases, and sentences by means of speech or writing.

The proliferation of language assessment protocols in the 1950s and 1960s saw three dramatic additions to the definition of aphasia. For example, Joseph Wepman (1951) specified that aphasia may be manifested as a breakdown in any or each of the four *language modalities:* listening or auditory comprehension, reading or visual comprehension, speaking or verbal expression, and writing or graphic expression. He also emphasized that aphasia was a consequence of cortical damage and distinguished it from factors implicating any faulty innervation of the musculature of speech (or dysarthria), dysfunction of the peripheral sense organs (blindness or deafness), or general mental deficiency. Hildred Schuell endorsed the specification of the four language modalities in aphasia definition and added that there may be variable degrees of impairment for each of the four modalities (Scheull, Jenkins & Jimenez-Pabon, 1964). Finally, Frank Benson highlighted the need for including linguistic/verbal features of aphasic communication through the determination of "fluent versus nonfluent" verbal output (Benson & Ardilla, 1996).

Each of the different historical contributions realizes the multiplicity of possible symptoms in aphasia and, therefore, implicates aphasia as a "syndrome." The available information is, therefore, reflected in the following characterization of the nature of aphasia:

- It is an acquired language disorder implying that the individual had normal language and communication skills at one time.
- It is a consequence of damage to the language processing parts of the brain, which establishes a neurological basis for the disorder.
- It may affect one or each of the four language modalities including auditory comprehension, reading comprehension, verbal expression, and written expression; the degree of disruption for each of the modalities may differ in severity.
- The related communication symptoms may demonstrate unique clusters or patterns in their presentation, which serve to identify different types (or classification) of aphasia.

COGNITIVE-COMMUNICATION DISORDERS

Cognition is an umbrella term that includes a variety of low (or simple) and high (or complex) order functions of the brain that typify an individual's survival, interaction, and self-preservation. *Cognitive disorder* refers to the difficulty in maintaining a logical and coherent flow of conversation, maintaining attention, and thinking on an abstract level. An impairment of even a select few of the myriad cognitive components can adversely affect communication. The term *cognitive-communication disorder* is used to denote a direct connection between the impaired cognitive function and the overt breakdown in communication. Cognitive-communication disorders are distinguishable because of the following factors:

- They are not restricted to focal, or circumscribed, lesions involving the dominant hemisphere exclusively.
- They may result from damage to the nondominant (right) hemisphere, or from diffused (nonfocal) head trauma, or even from multiple infarctions or lesion sites.
- A common link between the different forms of cognitive-communication disorders are the involvement of the prefrontal cortex and its connections with the limbic system.

LANGUAGE/LINGUISTIC SYMPTOMS

Historically, there have been some influencing descriptors that led to the characterization of linguistic symptoms in aphasia. For example, John Hughlings Jackson described aphasia as a loss of *propositional* (volitional or intentional) speech, which he distinguished from *subpropositional* speech representing automatic, overlearned and overused phrases such as social greetings, expletives, or rote/sequential counting. Kurt Goldstein (1942) elaborated this dichotomy to include the physiological sequelae of brain damage with the contention that the prevailing communication disorder is reflective of positive and negative symptoms. He attributed *positive symptoms* to isolation, or severation of the impaired and intact areas of the brain; while *negative symptoms* occurred because of the nonfunctioning damaged areas. Positive symptoms generally imply occurrences that are beyond normal expectations. Some examples of positive communication symptoms include the use of subpropositional speech, or misuse of words or phrases (errors); similarly, exaggerated motor reflexes or excessive muscle tone reflect positive motor symptoms, while agitation and hallucination characterize positive cognitive symptoms. Negative symptoms connote diminished performance. Examples of negative communication symptoms include the inability to comprehend instructions, inability to name objects or familiar persons, or nonfluent verbal output; examples of negative motor symptoms include paralysis of an arm, leg, or both (hemiplegia).

The observed positive and negative symptoms occur because of *diaschisis* which according to von Monakow, implies that functions of (nondamaged) areas that are remote from the location of damage may be suspended; thus cerebral edema, or the anatomical and physiological isolation of nondamaged areas may account for diaschisis and resulting positive and negative symptoms. The effect of diaschisis may last from days to weeks, and its fading away corresponds to gradual recovery/improvement in functions over a period of time immediately after the CVA.

Some of the language-specific symptoms are clearly distinguishable as either positive or negative symptoms while others do not comply with this dichotomy. This section describes some of the prominent symptoms that impede decoding and/or encoding language; these symptoms are also summarized in Table 6.1.

Auditory Comprehension problem is primarily a dysfunction of the dominant (left) temporal lobe (auditory cortex) involving Wernickes's area. This symptom is characterized as difficulty understanding spoken language either in the form of instructions or during conversation. This problem also results due to any disruption between the auditory cortex and the limbic system.

Visual Comprehension problem reflects impaired ability to understand written (visual) information. The underlying site of lesion for this symptom is not as specific as for auditory comprehension problem; it may involve the visual (occipital) cortex and its connections with the other three primary lobes within the dominant hemisphere. The problem may range from difficulty recognizing letters or words, or there may be difficulty understanding written sentences; such problems are frequently determined as *dyslexia* or *alexia* (reading disorder).

Paraphasia is a generic term introduced by Sigmund Freud that

Table 6.1. Symptoms Reflecting Language, Behavioral and Cognitive, and Sensory-Perceptual and Motor Impairments.

Language	Behavioral & Cognitive	Sensory-perceptual	Motor
Severe auditory comprehension problem (auditory verbal agnosia/word deafness)	Euphoria	Central/retrocochlear hearing loss	Hemiplegia (& hemiparesis)
	Increased egocentricity	Diplopia	
Mild/selective auditory comprehension			Ataxia
(semantic or syntactic comprehension problem)	Increased affectiveness/automatism	Nystagmus	Seizures
Reading comprehension problem	Emotional lability	Hemianopia: homonymous & heteronymous	Apraxia: limb, constructional, oral & verbal
	Inconsistent/fluctuating responses	Auditory agnosia	Dysarthria
Paraphasia: phonemic/literal, neologistic, & semantic/verbal	Increased frustration	Visual agnosia	
Anomia/dysnomia/word-retrieval problem (semantic paraphasia, anaphor, circumlocution)	Stimulus boundness	Amusia	
	Reduced attention span	Autotopagnosia	
Nonfluent verbal output	Impaired abstraction/executive functions	Prosopagnosia	

Table 6.1 – *Continued*

Language	Behavioral & Cognitive	Sensory-perceptual	Motor
Fluent verbal output	Social withdrawal	Anosognosia/hemispatial inattention	
Agrammatism/telegrammatism	Depression		
Paragrammatism	Catastrophic reaction		
Confabulation/verbal irrelevancy	Increased dependency		
Jargon: semantic/extended English & extended neologistic jargon	Perseveration		
Agraphia/dysgraphia (paragraphia)	Spatial-temporal disorientation		
	Acalculia/dyscalculia		
	Retrograde & anterograde amnesia		

refs to errors in word production. Typically three specific types of paraphasias are possible: phonemic, neologistic, and semantic. *Phonemic* (or *literal*) *paraphasia* represents mispronouncing part of a word, which is frequently identified as a phonological retrieval problem. The most common manifestations of phonemic paraphasia may be substitution of a sound/consonant or syllable (e.g., "classes" for "glasses"), or addition of an extraneous consonant or syllable (e.g., "biglasses" for "glasses"), or omission (deletion) of a consonant or syllable (e.g., "lasses" for "glasses," which also represents simplification of a blend). Research on phonemic paraphasia has shown that such errors tend to occur more often in pre-vocalic (preceding a vowel) positions and in stressed syllables within words perhaps because these consonant + vowel syllables tend to make a greater contribution toward word meaning. The data also indicate that fricative consonant groups (e.g., /s, z, f, v/) tend to evoke a greater number of phonemic paraphasias (Holloman & Drummond, 1991). *Neologistic paraphasia* is the use of a nonmeaningful or nonsense word. Although the word can be perceived as strings of familiar consonant syllables, it is not representative of a meaningful word (e.g., "teti"). Generally, those consonants that are easier to produce, and are frequently used in one's native language, tend to occur more often as neologistic paraphasia. This type of paraphasic production obviously causes a greater degree of communication disruption; their presence endorses the underlying phonological and/or semantic retrieval problem. Finally, *semantic* (or *verbal*) *paraphasia* represent word substitution errors and they are discussed later in this section.

Nonfluent versus *fluent verbal output* provides an insight into possible disruptions in the morphosyntactic components of verbal productions. The concept of verbal fluency was introduced in the 1860s however, its adaptation for clinical application did not occur until the 1970s. The distinction between nonfluent and fluent verbal output is summarized in Table 6.2. *Nonfluent verbal output* is typically associated with either focal or extensive lesions of the left (dominant) frontal lobe involving Broca's area. Verbal nonfluency may include some or each of the following features:

- Very limited quantity (or sparse) of verbal output.
- Average utterance length may be less than five words.
- Greater proportion of substantive (or content) than nonsubstantive (or function) words.

- Frequent omissions of grammatical morphemes (prefixes and suffixes).
- Production of incomplete or fragmented phrases and a limited variety of sentences.
- Slow, effortful and halting speaking rate (less than 50 words per minute).
- Excessive pausing between words and phrases.
- Flat speech intonation with minimal evidence of inflection within and across utterances.

The restricted length and complexity of utterances in nonfluent verbal output are identified as *agrammatism* (absence of grammar) or *telegrammatisms* (limited grammar). The obvious characterisitics of a/telegrammatisms are the disproportionate use of content words with parallel omission of grammatical words (e.g., "is," "are") and grammatical markers such as suffixes (e.g., "Boy *throw* ball" for "Boy *throws/is throwing* the ball"). The likelihood of omitting grammatical words and markers is greater if such words are unstressed in a sentence production; their deletion perhaps reflects a form of linguistic simplification (or compensation) strategy. This contention is verified through the observation that a nonfluent individual can use the grammatical morphemes if they are stressed to convey specific meanings (e.g., "Boy *is* (indeed) throwing the ball").

Fluent verbal output can be observed in normal individuals as well as in those with either mild or severe communication disorders. This type of verbal fluency is generally not associated with a specific lesion site; it may be observed in the presence of a nonspecific or diffuse lesion, or with extensive postrolandic left (dominant) hemispheric lesion, or even with subcortical lesions. Fluent verbal output implies the presence of some or all of the following features:

- Use of normal, or lengthy and complex sentence structures.
- Average utterance length is greater than five words.
- Greater or equal proportion of function than substantive (content) words.
- Presence of errors in use of grammatical morphemes.
- Rapid, or normal (noneffortful) speaking rate than may exceed 200 words per minute.
- Sufficient, or normal speech intonation and inflection.

Presence of any grammatical errors associated with fluent verbal out-

Table 6.2. Characterization of Nonfluent and Fluent Verbal Output in Aphasia.

Characteristics	Nonfluent Aphasia	Fluent Aphasia
Quantity of output	Limited/ sparse (fewer than 50 word per minute)	Normal (up to 200 words per minute)
Speaking effort	Increased (laborious) effort	Normal ease of speaking
Phrase/ utterance length (mean length of utterance)	Short utterances (1-2 word phrases)	Normal length (longer than 5 word phrases)
Speech prosody (stress, inflection and rate)	Dysprosodic (flat) output (slow rate and lacks inflection)	Normal/ rapid rate and inflection
Verbal content (content versus function words)	Excess of substantives (greater proportion of content words)	Lacks substantives (greater use of function words)
Grammatical morphemes	Frequent omissions (a/telegrammatism)	Erroneously used (paragrammatism)
Occurrence of paraphasias (phonemic, semantic, neologistic)	May vary in occurrence and types	Commonly observed

put is identified as *paragrammatism.* Such deviations may be represented as omission, addition or substitution of grammatical morphemes (e.g., "Boy is throwing the ball in [for "with"] the bat.")

Anomia, or *dysnomia* (naming problem) is the inability to access and use a word; it is commonly determined as *word finding* or *word retrieval problem.* Normally, the process of word/lexicon retrieval results from selection of precise sensory (visual, auditory, etc.), perceptual (common versus unique attributes), semantic (the thought to be conveyed), syntactic (how the word is to be used in an utterance), and phonetic (number and arrangement of syllables) features. Word retrieval problem is evident whenever brain function is compromised irrespective of any anatomical evidence of brain damage. It may also occur as a consequence of normal aging and in this context it is frequently described as the "tip-of-the-tongue" phenomenon. The severity of word retrieval problem is influenced by the size of brain damage, acuteness of the neurological dysfunction, and a variety of linguistic and perceptual variables. Although no one location is responsible for word retrieval, damage to areas within the dominant temporal (T2 and T3) and angular and supramarginal gyri are implicated whenever anomia is the exclusive problem.

Clinical manifestation of a word retrieval problem may be reflected through the occurrence of one or more of the following characteristics:

- *Semantic* (or *verbal) paraphasia* is a word substitution error where an incorrect word is used in place of the target item (e.g., "chair" for "table"). This manifestation implies that there was a constructive internal effort to recall the target word however, the outcome was not completely successful. The substituted word may share some perceptual, semantic, or phonological association with the target word; or the misused word may have no association with the target word.
- *Anaphors* are use of indefinite pronouns ("it") and word combinations ("that one, that thing") in place of the target word. The substitution of such vague words and phrases whenever the situation calls for retrieving a precise word reflects an evasive verbal strategy that is perhaps more challenging to modify during intervention.
- *Circumlocution,* or "beat around the bush," is observed when the individual resorts to sharing his/her knowledge or description of

the target lexicon if he is unable to provide its precise label. For example, instead of naming "table" the individual may say: "I have one too, one in the dining room and one for work."

Confabulation, or *verbal irrelevancy,* is the production of an off-target, or tangential, response that does not relate to the posed question. For example, the response to the posed question: "What is the woman doing?" may be "She seems to be spending a lot of time in the bedroom." Linguistically, such inappropriate productions are considered as a pragmatic problem. Sometimes they may be determined as topic-focus *disorganization/intersentential noncohesion* if they occur across consecutive utterances (e.g., "She had a baby . . . and then, I went out to eat."). It is important to note that confabulation or topic-focus disorganization can be identified only in the presence of fluent verbal output because it mandates increased quantity of verbal output, or *verbosity.*

Jargon simply refers to nonsense verbal productions that do not convey any meaning. If such nonmeaningful output utilizes strings of English words, then they are determined *semantic jargon* or *extended English jargon.* However, strings of non-English gibberish productions are determined *extended* (or *undifferentiated*) *neologism;* sometimes a true English word may be used within a cluster of extended neologism and such production is deemed *extended differentiated neologism.*

Agraphia, or *dysgraphia,* refers to difficulty expressing oneself through written language. The level of difficulty may range from total inability to write or the presence of errors in written output, also known as *paragraphia.* Paragraphia is an umbrella term that encompasses word spelling errors, grammatical errors, and word usage errors.

SENSORY AND PERCEPTUAL SYMPTOMS

Problems with recognition and perception of sensory signals via the two primary modalities, auditory and visual, are frequently associated with brain (CNS) damage. Sensory problems result if the receptor cells within the eye or ear are unable to convert a visual, or auditory, input to the designated electrical signal and transmit the signal to the brain via the respective cranial nerve. Sensory impairments are not generally associated with CNS lesions unless there is damage to the subcortical brainstem structures that are the first recipients of an incoming sensory message. Some examples of such auditory and visual sensory problems include the following:

- Central or retrocochlear hearing loss is associated with either cortical or subcortical lesions. There are reports of prevalence of high frequency (4 KHz and above) loss in diffused brain damage. The presence of such hearing loss can exacerbate prevailing listening and speech comprehension problems.
- *Diplopia,* or double vision can result from subcortical lesions at the level of midbrain and pons where the nerves responsible for ocular (eyeball) movements exit the brain. This symptom may interfere with recognition of objects and words.
- *Nystagmus* involves constant, rhythmic shifting movements of the eye that is associated with vestibular or cerebellar lesions; this impairment may disrupt visual processing as well.

Perception is defined as the processing and interpretation of sensory information; the interpretation results with the assistance of input from different sensory modalities, and thus perception operates as a "system." Any impairment in perception indicates an impaired ability to recognize and discriminate a stimulus from others and it is frequently determined as an agnosia. The term *agnosia* was introduced by Freud to denote impaired "gnosis" or awareness. Agnosia may result from right or left hemisphere lesions involving the primary sensory cortices (occipital, temporal, and parietal lobes), their interconnections with each other, and their subcortical pathways. The presence of agnosia may indeed interfere with communication and daily activities. Some examples of auditory perceptual problems include the following agnosias:

- *Auditory agnosia* can occur in lesions involving the primary auditory cortex (Heschl's gyrus in T1) of either the left or the right hemisphere; the lesion is generally anterior to Wernicke's area if it occurs in the dominant hemisphere. For example, the person verifies hearing a ringing sound and is able to localize the sound, but may not identify the nature of the sound by distinguishing it as either a door bell or a telephone ring.
- *Auditory verbal agnosia,* sometimes known as *pure word deafness,* specifies the breakdown in perceiving the significance of spoken words. This problem is also associated with severe auditory comprehension problem where the individual has difficulty recogniz-

ing similarities and differences between spoken words or following simple verbal instructions. This breakdown in auditory verbal
processing explains the presence of paraphasias, paragrammatisms, or semantic jargon in the victim's verbal output. Research
on dichotic listening (simultaneous auditory stimulation presented to both ears) during the 1960s has established left hemispheric dominancy for recognizing linguistic symbols such as numbers,
words and phrases. This finding implies that auditory verbal
agnosia results from damage to the language-dominant hemisphere involving the primary auditory area, planum temporale
and Wernicke's area and therefore, it is associated with extensive
lesions of the left temporal lobe involving the superior (T1) and
middle (T2) temporal gyri.

- *Amusia* refers to impaired perception of subtle tonal (prosodic)
features particularly relating to pitch. Its presence is verified
through the inability to detect the difference between familiar
songs containing slightly dissonant notes and the same songs
played in key. During speech perception, this problem may be
inferred if there is a breakdown in the ability to detect syllable or
word stressing however, individuals with amusia can discriminate
pitch inflections for spoken sentences versus questions. This
symptom may result from a dysfunction in the right temporal-
parietal region.

Several types of visual sensory-perceptual impairments may also be
associated with brain damage:

- *Hemianop(s)ia,* or impaired ability to detect objects in one-half of
the visual field, can occur when the optic pathways at the base of
the brain are involved. Several types of hemianopias are possible.
A *homonymous hemianopia* can occur if there is any disruption to
the optic tract or to the visual pathway between the optic chiasm
and the thalamus; there is impaired perception of objects in the
nasal and temporal fields on the same (right or left) side in this
condition. For example, damage to the left optic tract may result
in right homonymous hemianopia where objects in the right temporal and left nasal fields may not be perceived. A *heteronymous
hemianopia,* also known as *bitemporal hemianopia,* can occur if there
is any disruption at the optic chiasm; the resulting symptom is
deemed "tunnel vision" where objects placed in the nasal field are

recognized but those in the extreme/temporal (right or left) visual fields may not be perceived. There may also be *upper,* or *lower, quadrantic (homonymous) hemianopia* if one of the four visual field quadrants is involved; in such instances some of the optic radiation fibers to the occipital lobe may be damaged. Each of these possibilities is depicted in Figure 6-1.

- *Visual Agnosia* is the impaired recognition and differentiation of visual features relating to objects, shapes, or colors. It may be observed with either right or left hemisphere lesions involving the occipital lobe, or when the connections between the thalamus and the visual cortex (via the optic radiations) are compromised. The individual can see the presence of an object but is unable to identify its significance. Clinically, the presence of visual agnosia may exacerbate reading and writing problems and resultant errors are determined as alexia/dyslexia or agraphia/paragraphia, respectively.

- *Autotopagnosia* refers to the breakdown in the ability to recognize one's own body parts; it is also a manifestation of confusion between the right and left halves of the body. This form of agnosia is associated with cortical lesions in the right hemisphere, or with bilateral or diffuse cerebral lesions.

- *Prosopagnosia* is the impaired recognition of familiar faces and/or facial features and expressions. The individual may have difficulty distinguishing facial expressions depicting various emotions (e.g., happy, sad); or there may be confusion in differentiating familiar faces (e.g., sibling versus popular political leader or actor). This symptom is associated with right parietal lesions.

- *Anosognosia,* or *hemispatial inattention* (or unilateral "visual neglect") is also associated with right parieto-occipital lesions and sometimes including the temporal lobe as well. The individual with this condition tends to ignore the paralyzed (left) side; for example, the person may shave only the right side of the face. Severe patients may not even recognize their own body parts (autotopagnosia) and deny the diseased (paralyzed) condition. Generally, anosognosia is a transient symptom, which may subside within weeks following the brain injury.

Finally, *astereognosia,* or tactile agnosia, reflects an impaired ability to recognize an object exclusively via the sense of touch. This problem is

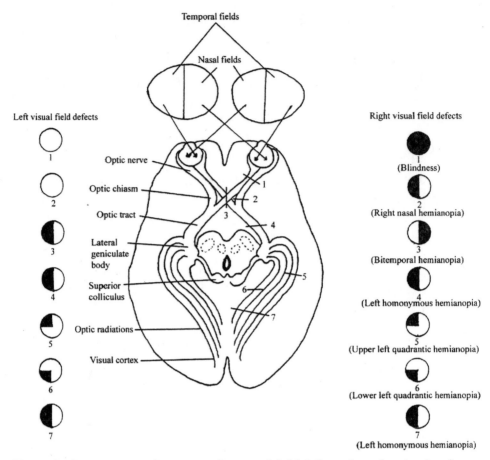

Figure 6.1. Lesion sites and corresponding visual field defects along the visual pathway.

confirmed if the individual can visually recognize an object but may not be able to do so with eyes closed.

BEHAVIORAL AND COGNITIVE SYMPTOMS

Behaviors are overt manifestations that describe an individual's response to a stimulus. A variety of behaviors that do not correspond to the patient's premorbid interaction style may be identified as a consequence of brain damage. The presence of such behaviors is noted if they interfere with efficient communication. Their occurrence is not confined to any specific lesion site or etiology; perhaps they are manifestations of cerebral edema or the effect of diaschisis, or even a learned coping strategy. The observed behavioral symptoms tend to complement, and sometimes exacerbate, accompanying cognitive impairments.

Cognitivism reflects an individual's ability to acquire and store information for self-preservation and survival. This aspect of brain function also plays an important role in combining old with recently acquired information to lead to new types of learning and behavior. Any disruption in underlying cognitive mechanisms can be reflected as overt behavioral symptoms. Clinically, an observed behavior can be considered abnormal if it is too frequent or excessive in its occurrence, or if it is inappropriate to the situation. Behavioral symptoms can be observed in routine interactions and thus they obviously contribute to communication problems as well. The following are some examples of behavioral-cognitive symptoms:

- *Euphoria,* sometimes referred as affective inappropriateness, is displayed as an overall sense of well-being, which may be displayed through the individual's rejection of any external input/feedback regarding the medical condition or management. For example, the patient may respond with "there is nothing wrong with my speech" when asked to complete a speech exercise. This behavior is seen in acute stages following brain lesion or surgery, and it can impede the recovery progress because of poor compliancy.

- *Increased egocentricity* can surface through the refusal to respond to a stimulus or situation that is not of interest or does not pertain to the individual's lifestyle. For example, the patient may refuse to name a common object if it is not in the person's repertoire; in extreme cases there may be selective difficulty using phrases that include the word "you or your."

- *Excessive affective* (or *automatic*) *behavior* can be observed through inappropriate and frequent verbal cursing or nonverbal (self-manipulation) behaviors. Such behaviors are subpropositional in nature and the individual may not be able to volitionally suppress them.

- *Emotional lability* is identified when inappropriate and excessive, or uncontrollable, release of emotions such as crying or laughter occurs with minimal provocation. For example, uninhibited crying because of person's inability to provide a response. Sometimes excessive release of laughter to an innocuous stimulus can turn to crying because the patient is cognizant of its inappropriateness and is embarrassed at the inability to regulate this behavior. The best management approach is to assure the patient that the symptom is partly due to the brain dysfunction and that he/she will gradually learn to overcome its occurrence. The clinician should not ignore the event because it increases the embarrassment for the patient and leads to adverse or poor rehabilitation outcome.

- *Inconsistent* or *fluctuating responses* to the same stimulus across different situations and times are frequently observed by family members and caregivers. Physiologically, such observations reflect the brain's coping and readjustment to the severed neural connections and the parallel healing process through the formation of alternate pathways. Inconsistent responses may also increase due to external factors such as task difficulty or fatigue, and to a challenging situation or communication partner.

- *Stimulus boundness* is observed when the individual's responses fixate on selective attributes of presented stimuli. This behavior is observed typically during the acute stages of recovery from brain damage. For example, elicited responses reflect exclusive focus on personal preferences or dislike of stimuli, or partiality toward select perceptual features (size or color) of the stimuli. This behavioral tendency is perhaps indicative of the individual's attempt at simplifying the demands of an abstract task.

- *Increased frustration* level when encountering difficulty in routine and simple situations is observed as a consequence of brain damage. This behavior also surfaces possibly due to the effect of physiological fatigue or the inability to handle a failure to respond.

- *Reduced attention span,* or acquired attention deficit, is identified if the individual has obvious difficulty maintaining focus on a structured task or a topic during conversation. The presence of this symptom is attributed to several endogenous and exogenous factors such as the effect of medication, fatigue, lack of interest in the presented task or topic, and underlying memory disorders.

- *Increased concretism,* or *reduced abstraction,* reflects impaired problem-solving abilities; this symptom is also described as *impaired executive function.* The broad characteristics include impairment in planning, reasoning and decision-making abilities. Clinically, the patient may have difficulty explaining similarities and differences between concepts, plan and organize thoughts and events and execute them in a methodical manner, derive at inductive and deductive reasoning, and perform simple calculations. Abstraction problems may be manifested differently in left versus right hemisphere lesions. For example, a left-hemisphere damaged patient may see the overall theme of an action or event in a picture but not be able to link the different components to each other; while the right-hemisphere damaged patient perceives the details relating to the different constituents but cannot formulate the theme of the picture.

- *Social withdrawal* may occur in some situations because the individual may not be able to cope with the visual and auditory ambiences in certain environments. For example, the person may no longer enjoy mingling with people in a crowded or noisy room following the brain damage.
- *Depression* is identified in approximately 30–50 percent of individuals with brain damage, and more often in chronic stages (6 months to 2 years) after the damage. This symptom is generally associated with lesions of the left frontal lobe involving the prefrontal cortex and its connections. Depression may be exacerbated by other factors as well, including slower gains/recovery, unrealistic self-expectations, premorbid personality, and insidious biochemical changes in the brain.
- *Catastrophic reaction* is an excessive and inappropriate reaction to a "routine" stimulus, task or situation. It may be precipitated by intrinsic factors such as increased frustration from failure or fatigue, unable to rationalize or shift focus from the difficult situation, and vascular changes in the brain. A catastrophic reaction may be manifested as a seizure event, inappropriate and sudden onset of rage, or emotional lability. Occasionally, external factors such as persistent prodding to continue a difficult activity may precipitate the catastrophic behavior. Some management options include taking a short break from the task, or switch to a general conversation or an easier task, or even terminate the session.
- *Increased dependency* behavior is typically fostered by the spouse/caregiver or the attending clinician who tend to be conciliatory and overanticipate/meet the patient's needs. Such "overcaring" can impede recovery if the patient is not encouraged to make independent responses or decisions pertaining to his/her personal needs.

- *Perseveration,* or intrusion phenomenon, is the inability to shift from a previously appropriate response to a newer one; it is an inappropriate occurrence of a prior response after an intervening stimulus. For example, the patient may get stuck on naming a series of unrelated pictures as "dog" even though the earlier-presented picture of a dog has been withdrawn. Perseveration may occur across consecutive responses or they may occur after up to 20 minutes following the initial response. Frequently used words are most likely to be perseverated, and the individual may perseverate on either an accurate or inaccurate response. The presence of verbal perseveration is also influenced by the linguistic context; it is observed more often during sentence completion and naming tasks, and less often in word reading tasks. Possible management strategies include reduced rate of stimulus presentation, and use of greater pauses between consecutive responses tend to reduce the occurrences of perseveration.
- *Disorientation* is manifested as the inability to provide information regarding place (spatial disorientation) or time (temporal disorientation). For example, the patient may be unable to recognize that he/she is in the hospital, or distinguish between nighttime versus daytime.
- *Acalculia* (or *dyscalculia*) refers to calculation problems where the individual cannot perform the four basic arithmetic processes: addition, subtraction, multiplication, or division. Sometimes this problem is considered an overt manifestation of an underlying abstraction problem. In severe instances, the individual may be unable to recognize, count and copy numbers.
- *Amnesia* is impairment in memory implicating disrupted ability to store sensory information for later retrieval as images, thoughts and ideas. Memory is a primary requirement for learning and is therefore, an important cognitive function. Amnesia associated with dysfunction of the hippocampus and its complex interconnections with the surrounding tissue including the rhinal cortex, amygdala, parts of diencephalon (medial thalamus and mammillary bodies), medial temporal lobe, and orbital prefrontal cortex. Thus, amnesia may reflect itself in many forms: there may be dysfunction of memories dependent on emotions and olfaction, as well as those dependent on visuospatial and auditory experiences. The two common types of amnesia are anterograde and retro-

grade amnesia. *Anterograde amnesia* is the impaired ability to form new memories or learn new information. The person lives in "eternal present" and cannot form factual memories such as remembering what happened a few minutes ago; such an individual may forget new instructions or assignments but can recall old memories. In contrast, *retrograde amnesia* is the condition when the individual cannot recover previous (long-term) memories particularly those relating to recollecting special events in his/her life (e.g., events relating to one's wedding). Such problems in recalling autobiographical memories are associated with medial temporal lobe lesions.

MOTOR SYMPTOMS

This section describes some of the physical or motor consequences of brain damage. The presence of these symptoms may depend on factors such as the extent and location of brain damage, as well as the recency of the damage. Persistent motor deficits are sometimes considered the primary indicators for rehabilitation because of their influence on accomplishing routine/daily activities.

- *Hemiplegia* implies the inability to move, or has paralysis of, one-half side of the body; usually the side opposite (*contralateral*) the damaged hemisphere is paralyzed. For example, in case of a left hemispheric lesion involving the precentral gyrus and its subcortical connections, there is paralysis of the right side of the body. It needs to be noted that there is no significant clinical relationship between the presence of hemiplegia and severity of aphasia. Sometimes there may be paralysis of any one limb, or *monoplegia*. It is rare for a cortical lesion to result in *paraplegia* where the two lower limbs are paralyzed; this condition, however, is generally associated with lower spinal cord lesions. Occasionally, a patient with combined cortical and subcortical/brainstem lesion may have *quadriplegia* if all four limbs are paralyzed. Each of these problems are different from *alternating hemiplegia* where there is an ipsilateral paralysis of one side of face and tongue with simultaneous paralysis of the contralateral extremities. Here the lesion is subcortical in nature, but it is above the *decussation* (crossover) of the descending pyramidal tracts in the medulla.

- *Hemiparesis* is weakening of muscle functions on one-half side of the body; it implies that the motor movement is below par, but not totally paralyzed.
- *Ataxia* refers to disturbance in balance or inability to coordinate motor movements, which may resemble a drunken state. This symptom is associated with cerebellar or vestibular dysfunction and their connections with the brainstem; there is no obvious motor or sensory disability.
- *Contractures* refers to stiffening of muscles due to excessive spasticity or nonuse, is also associated with limb paralysis. This condition exacerbates the motor limitations and recovery from rehabilitation.
- *Seizures* represent electrical storms in the cortex due to increased activation of the neurons surrounding the damaged area. Sometimes old scars from previous brain damage can also create short circuits to result in seizure activity; they can also be triggered by excessive fatigue. The target origins that cause seizures can be detected via round the clock EEGs. Seizures are generally controlled by medication when they occur as a consequence of the brain damage. If seizures occur during a therapy session, they should be managed by removing obstacles such as furniture to prevent the patient from additional trauma; the precipitating factor(s), duration, and type of seizure activity should also be noted and it is advisable to discontinue the activity or the session in the event of a seizure.

Lesions involving the motor cortex primarily results in motor programming (or planning) problems, and these are grouped as *apraxia,* or *dyspraxia.* Apraxia may result from either right or left cortical lesions, and they are generally associated with lesions involving the frontal lobe and its connections with the occipital and/or parietal lobes. There is no paresis or paralysis of the muscles; the primary problem involves inappropriate completion of sequential motor acts. Another characteristic of apraxia is the discrepancy in performing volitional and automatic movements; the body part may not complete the motor act under command/voluntary control, but it can accomplish the same movement involuntarily. The following are some examples of commonly reported apraxias:

- *Limb* or *motor apraxia* is identified when there is disorganized (impaired) object use. For example, when asked to show the use

of a cigarette, the patient may hold it as a pencil.
- *Constructional apraxia* relates to disrupted ability to reconstruct a design with three-dimensional blocks, or there is an inability to copy or draw a design. This impaired function is associated with right parietal lobe lesions.
- *Oral apraxia,* also known as *buccofacial apraxia,* may result from frontal lobe lesions in either hemisphere. The patient is unable to voluntarily imitate oral sequential (diadochokinetic) movements with the lips and tongue, but may be able to do so involuntarily as when eating.
- *Verbal apraxia,* or *apraxia of speech,* is the impaired ability to perform sequential speech movements. The breakdown may be exacerbated when producing longer words (multiple syllables), and the observed verbal errors may be described as phonemic paraphasias as well. Verbal apraxia may occur concurrently with Broca's aphasia in the presence of extensive left frontal lobe lesions.

Finally, lesions of the primary motor strip (precentral gyrus) and associated subcortical, efferent pathways involving either hemisphere can result in speech production problems, or *dysarthria.* Unlike formulation of expressive language, or sequencing speech syllables as in verbal apraxia, dysarthria is a consequence of disrupted outgoing (descending) signals along the motor pathways within and outside the CNS. Consequently, the individual is unable to move target muscles in a smooth and coordinated fashion; the impaired movements are observed during both voluntary and involuntary motor acts. Fundamentally, dysarthria results in impaired/reduced speech intelligibility (or understandability) due to the inefficient movement of the vocal tract structures. The term *anarthria* is used if there is total inability to move the muscles that are necessary for speech production; this problem is typically identified in bilateral lower brainstem lesions.

OTHER SYMPTOMS

There is one other symptom, *bowel* and *bladder incontinency,* that needs to be mentioned since it has some relevance to the rehabilitation team. This problem can occur due to two possible factors:
- Cerebral edema, which may increase fluid secretion and/or gen-

eral confusion or disorientation.

• Purposeful manipulation, where the patient may provoke (or stage) the biological need to void as a reason to be excused or withdraw from a situation or caregiver.

SUMMARY

The syndrome of aphasia and cognitive-communication disorders is analogous to a kaleidoscope with the possibility of observing a collage of symptoms that occur in combinations unique to a given patient. The symptoms may be categorized according to linguistic, behavioral, cognitive and sensory-perceptual domains however just like the colors and shapes of the image in a kaleidoscope can change with a gentle shake, the groupings of select clinical/communication symptoms can differ between brain-damaged individuals. Table 6.3 provides the schemata of the neurological basis for the different communication-related functions. This depiction is an attempt to emphasize the inter-relationship between neuroanatomy (structures and levels), neuro-physiology (functions) and corresponding symptoms resulting from their disruption.

Successful determination of the dominant symptoms should be the primary clinical pursuit of all clinicians. This outcome is possible through an understanding of the symptoms, possible co-occurrence of select symptoms, and clinical vigilance and intuition. This journey to knowledge acquisition is a challenging process but once this skill is acquired, the decisions regarding management and rehabilitation are relatively obvious.

Table 6.3. Neurological Substrate for Linguistic-Communication Functions and Corresponding Symptoms.

(Cortical Region)

	Sensory Cortex	Sensory+Association Cortex	Limbic System	All lobes	Motor Cortex
	Temporal, parietal, occipital lobes	(Wernicke's area)	Limbic lobe, insula, prefrontal cortex & subcortical connections	(Broca's area)	Frontal lobe: motor strip
Functions	Perception/ discrimination (auditory, visual, tactile)	Comprehension (decoding) (auditory, visual)	Memory (short & long term) Executive functions	Production (encoding) Speech	Praxis Voluntary motor mvmnt
Symptoms	Agnosias: auditory, visual, tactile	Aphasia: comprehension problems Word deafness Alexia	Higher order cognitive problems Acalculia Confabulation (irrelevancy)	Aphasia: nonfluent/fluent Tele-/paragrammatism Jargon Paraphasias Agraphia (&paragraphia)	Apraxia: oral, limb Dysarthria Hemiplegia

Subcortical Region
Diencephalon & reticular formation

Functions
Attention
Perception
Orientation

Symptoms
Low order cognitive problems
Hemianopias

Subcortical Region
Corpus striatum, cerebellum

Functions
Voluntary & involuntary mvmnt
Motor coordination
Automatic behaviors

Symptoms
Dyskinesia
Dysarthria

Table 6.3 – *Continued*

Subcortical Region
(CN sensory nuclei & rhombencephalic reticular formation)

Functions
Arousal
Sensation

Symptoms
Blindness
Diplopia
Hearing loss

Subcortical Region
Brainstem: CN motor nuclei

Functions
Motor movements
Reflexive behaviors

Symptoms
Dysarthria
Ipsilateral paralysis

Chapter 7

ASSESSMENT OF COMMUNICATION AND RELATED FUNCTIONS

Assessment implies documenting the presence, or absence, of a disorder and corresponding clinical manifestations. Its goal is to determine possible management options to alleviate or minimize the clinical symptoms. The assessment process also helps identify individuals who may, or may not, optimally benefit from rehabilitation. The format for an assessment protocol depends on the clinical purpose and urgency for making decisions regarding diagnosis, recommendations and management.

TEST SELECTION

The rationale and selection of an appropriate test protocol results from the following considerations:

- The assessment goal is to merely detect the presence or absence of possible breakdown in communication; in this instance, a "screening" protocol is generally performed.
- The time constraint, or need for expediency, in making a diagnosis may influence the assessment decision; brief test batteries may be considered as appropriate under such conditions to help identify the primary areas of deficits.
- Patients at early/acute stages following the brain damage may be clinically unstable or may not be able to tolerate lengthy and highly structured diagnostic tests. Their tendency to show fluctuating performances, readily fatiguing, or they may improve rapidly which may justify the use of brief test batteries.

119

- The extent of the brain damage is also a major consideration when selecting an assessment protocol. Again, a brief testing procedure may be sufficient to help identify the degree of the communication problem and the prevailing communication-enhancing capabilities.
- The need to identify specific areas of impairment or verify the presence of select symptoms may call for use of detailed and comprehensive protocol. Comprehensive test batteries tend to be lengthier in administration and therefore, they are generally used with physiologically stable patients.
- The attempt to understand a possible relationship between observed performance and corresponding site of lesion information may call for use of esoteric tests however, they can be time-consuming as well.
- The determination of candidacy for referral and potential for recovery and rehabilitation may dictate the use of select assessments; such tests focus on evaluating possible strengths or facilitators that enhance communication performance.
- Evaluation of progress from intervention may be performed through structured tests and in nonstructured social situations. The selected protocol should help determine the degree of improvement or compensation of functions to establish discharge planning and community re-entry decisions.

Some of the frequently used test protocols for assessing different components of communication are listed at the end of the chapter (see Appendix A). Of these, the language screening and comprehensive language tests are used primarily to evaluate the presence, severity and type of aphasia, while those listed under supplementary tests and functional communication assessment can be used to assess any individual with brain damage.

There are four essential ingredients for considering a diagnostic instrument. They include provision of a valid rationale, its design and description, its scoring and interpretation, and related standardization information. The test *rationale* should specify its purpose, whether it aims to detect the presence or absence of a disorder, or if its goal is to provide a comprehensive characterization of the nature of the disorder and related symptoms. For example, the criterion-related validity of a test instrument is verified through its ability to discriminate normal from deviant performance. The depth of a test is closely associated to its purpose; thus some tests are brief while others are relatively lengthy and detailed. Some protocols are appropriate for either acute or for chronic patients, and some may link the observed performances to a theoretical language or neurological model. Irrespective of these factors, the test should reflect consistency in its *design* and *organization* through the following features:

- Stimulus adequacy (number), diversity (objects, pictures, letters and words), attributes (grammatical and semantic category), and familiarity (frequency of use)
- Delineation of specific subtests (tasks) for the four language modalities (auditory and visual comprehension, verbal and written expression)
- Task organization should demonstrate some form of hierarchy, either progressing from easy to difficult tasks or vice versa.

Each of these components strengthens the content and construct validity of the selected tool.

Test *administration* and *scoring* procedures should strive for inter- and intraexaminer reliability. Its utilization of the "stimulus-response" matrix fosters specification of instructions for stimulus presentation and corresponding response elicitation and scoring. The parameters for scoring elicited responses should be obvious whether it utilizes accuracy criteria, rating scales, response times, or cues. Response *interpretation* should help formulate an impression regarding severity and/or classification of the disorder. It should also highlight the symptoms that contribute to the disorder, help identify similarities and differences in performances across modalities and subtest areas, and also permit observations regarding possible facilitators or obstructive behaviors. Each of these considerations attests to the stability of a test as demonstrated through its *standardization.* The sum effect of the four aspects of a test help establish the "sensibility" of an assessment protocol in terms of its importance, reasonableness, and ease of use; these factors ultimately influence the success or failure of a clinical measurement.

COMPONENTS OF STANDARD LANGUAGE ASSESSMENT

The typical language examination protocol assesses the four language modalities with more than one level of competency being evaluated within each modality. Although such protocols are commonly used to diagnose aphasia, they are also used for individuals with cognitive-communication disorders. The available tests may either serve as screening protocols or they provide comprehensive battery of information (see Appendix A).

Some common tasks within each of the four language modalities, and clinical inferences that can be made from assessing them are listed in Table 7.1; these tasks have been summarized from available aphasia examination tests. Of the four language modalities, those relating to auditory comprehension and verbal expression are prioritized since the acts of listening and speaking are fundamentals for human communication. A sample language screening protocol is also provided in Appendix B.

AUDITORY (LISTENING) COMPREHENSION: The selected tasks within this modality evaluate the proficiency of listening skills for understanding spoken language. Generally, this modality is assessed first, and its tasks are presented in a hierarchical order to progress from relatively easy to more challenging tasks ranging from matching and pointing (discrimination) to answering (yes/no) questions, following lengthy commands and understanding narrative text. The tasks assessing this modality are so designed that they require little or no verbal response, which help maintain focus on the goal to evaluate the degree of listening difficulty (see Table 7.1). The stimuli are also selected to assess the influence of type, length and grammatical complexity on auditory processing ability. This consideration is based on the contention that the efficiency of listening skills decreases as the demands from these stimuli increase; therefore, stimulus characteristics can help distinguish the nature and severity of the comprehension problem as well. During this initial phase of assessment, any bias toward select stimulus items may be identified as well. For example, an individual with increased egocentricity may fail to "Point to the stove" if the person is unfamiliar to the depiction of a "wood stove," but this person may encounter no difficulty recognizing a contemporary/familiar kitchen stove. Sometimes a single stimulus can be used to evaluate several different abilities: identification of body parts ("Point to your *eyes*"), follow simple commands ("Close your *eyes*"), or axial commands ("Point to your left *eye*").

VERBAL (ORAL) EXPRESSION: This modality assesses verbal proficiency and ease of speech production; it also provides an estimate

Table 7.1. Components of Standard Language Assessment and Possible Clinical Symptoms Accounting for Difficulty Completing the Different Tasks/Areas.

Modalities and Subtest Areas	Examples of Tasks	Possible Contributing Symptoms (deficits)
Auditory (listening) comprehension		
Recognition/discrimination	Recognize/match sounds or words	Auditory agnosia/auditory verbal agnosia
	Identify body parts ("Point to your eye")	Severe comprehension problem; autotopagnosia
Understand simple instruction	Identify common objects and pictures	Comprehension problem; visual agnosia
	Identify colors and shapes	Comprehension problem; visual agnosia
	Follow single commands ("Close the window")	Comprehension problem; visual agnosia
	Follow axial commands ("Point to your left eye.")	Comprehension problem; visual/auto- topagnosia
Understand longer/complex information	Follow 2 and 3 step commands ("Close the window, turn off the lights and sit down")	Mild (syntactical) comprehension & STM problems
	Answer "Yes/No" questions ("Is grass green?")	Mild comprehension and STM problems
	Paragraph/story retention (assess via "yes/no" questions)	Mild (syntactical) comprehension & STM problems
Verbal (oral) expression		
Repetition	Repeat single to polysyllabic words ("Say the word . . .")	Verbal apraxia; STM problem; phonemic paraphasia
	Repeat short and long, familiar & unfamiliar phrases	Verbal apraxis; telegrammatism
Word Retrieval	Convergent naming (objects, pictures, body parts, colors)	Anomia; possible agnosias; verbal apraxia
	Divergent naming (number of animals or foods named)	Anomia; STM problem; verbal apraxia
	Sequential naming (numbers 1–10 or days of week)	LTM problems; dysprosody
Automatic speech	Recite rhyme ("Jack and Jill"); sing ("Happy birthday")	LTM problems; dysprosody

Table 7.1 – *Continued*

Modalities and Subtest Areas	Examples of Tasks	Possible Contributing Symptoms (deficits)
Self-expression (connected speech)	Open-ended conversation (favorite vacation) Describe picture or a procedure (cook an egg/change tire)	Nonfluent/fluent; anomia; verbal apraxia; telegrammatism/paragrammtism; verbal irrelevancy/confabulation
Oral Diadochokinesis	Perform nonspeech movements ("open-close mouth 5 times") Perform speech movements ("Say butter 5 times")	Oral apraxia; comprehension & STM problems Oral &/verbal apraxia; comprehension & STM prob.
Visual (reading) comprehension		
Recognition/discrimination	Match pictures, letters, colors, or shapes	Visual agnosia; hemianopia; dyslexia
Word comprehension/recognition	Match words; identify misspelled words	Literacy; Visual agnosia; hemianopia; dyslexia
Understand simple sentences	Match phrases; match sentence-to-picture	Dyslexia; comprehension problem
Understand complex information	Paragraph (silent) reading (assess via multiple choice)	Dyslexia; comprehension and STM problems
Written (graphic) expression		
Eye-hand coordination	Copy name, numbers, letters or words	Hemianopia; agraphia (paragraphia); LTM and STM problems; literacy issues
Simple writing	Write words or simple phrases to dictation	STM problems; literacy issues
Self-expression	Describe a picture in narrative writing	STM problems; literacy issues
Other		
Combined reading and verbal production	Oral (outloud) word/sentence reading	Any/all visual or oral symptoms
Abstract reasoning/calculation	Complete simple addition and subtraction problems	Acalculia; impaired executive functions

of residual communication capability. The efficiency of spoken language is assessed through five broad areas: word and sentence repetition, word retrieval, automatic/sequential speech, connected speech proficiency, and oral motor skills. Repetition of spoken words and phrases are typically controlled for features such as length and familiarity of the stimuli. Word retrieval is assessed through two types of naming tasks: *convergent* naming requires the recall of the exact name of the stimulus presented as either an object, picture, number or body part, and related tasks are administered through picture/object naming or sentence completions. In contrast, *divergent* naming permits self-generated recall of as many names representing a target semantic category; this format evaluates the number of items retrieved, their accuracy/appropriateness, and the time taken to retrieve them. Divergent naming tasks are also termed word fluency or word generation tasks. Automatized speech perhaps aims to assess subpropositional speech by requiring the provision of overlearned information such as sequential naming of numbers, days of week, or recitation of nursery rhymes and popular songs. The rationale for using a variety of naming tasks relates to the fact that lexicon learning and retrieval is dependent on a variety of sensory-perceptual systems including visual, auditory, tactile, olfactory, etc.

Connected speech elicitation utilizes the divergent format by indulging in either an open-ended conversation with the patient, or requiring the patient to describe action-depicting pictures, or provide a verbal monologue by sharing a memorable event or action-oriented procedure. This context is clinically challenging because it helps determine several possible symptoms and their interactions. For example, it may ascertain the nature of verbal fluency (nonfluent or fluent), word retrieval problem (anomia), concurrent neuromuscular problem (dysarthria), verbal apraxia, STM or LTM problems, different types of paraphasia, telegrammatism versus paragrammatism, as well as verbal irrelevancies and confabulations. Finally, oral motor proficiency is demonstrated through the ability to move the lips and tongue across successive trials. Related tasks evaluate nonspeech and speech diadochokinetic, or alternating movements between two opposing positions (see Table 7.1). Sometimes these movements are observed during vegetative (e.g., licking, smacking) and voluntary acts to verify any inconsistencies between related motor movements; such comparison can confirm the presence of concurrent speech disorders such as dysarthria, and oral or verbal apraxia. This component evaluates possible influence of the subcortical neuromotor pathways and target muscles on oral (language) expression as well.

VISUAL (READING) COMPREHENSION: This modality focuses on the ability to recognize objects and symbols that are presented visually. Similar to auditory comprehension, the tasks may represent a hierarchical order, progressing from relatively easier to more challenging responses (see Table 7.1). The presented stimuli may need to be adjusted if there is a concern regarding literacy and premorbid reading competency. Clinically, the presented tasks estimate possible visual perceptual (agnosia or hemianopia) or comprehension (dyslexia) problems, as well as visual retention (STM) problems. Assessment of this modality also substantiates any bias toward, or against, any stimuli that were identified during the assessment of other modalities. For example, a comparison of responses between silent and oral (out loud) reading may help determine if the impaired reading performance is influenced by the oral expression modality or if it is an exclusive manifestation of a visual processing problem.

GRAPHIC (WRITING) EXPRESSION: The tasks within this modality evaluate prerequisite motor skills for eye-hand coordination, as well as the ability to formulate written language to determine if the observed residual skills can augment the aphasic individual's verbal limitations. Again, the tasks and stimuli represent some hierarchical organization (see Table 7.1); the assessment of this modality may also call for a modification in task presentation if there is any concern regarding literacy or visual-motor problems. Elicited responses obviously help infer the proficiency of residual writing skills for self-expression/communication; they also evaluate any interference from visual field, comprehension and word-finding problems. Written responses can also endorse the influence of short and/or long-term recall problems.

OTHER AREAS: In addition to oral reading tasks, simple arithmetic tasks are sometimes included in assessment to determine problems in abstraction or executive functions. Of course, any difficulty encountered during the presented calculation tasks is deemed acalculia (see Table 7.1). Sometimes peripheral sensory functions such as visual and auditory acuity, and neuromuscular integrity through speech intelligibility, are frequently included in a communication assessment protocol as well. Screening for visual acuity is performed when there are obvious signs of diplopia, hemianopia or visual agnosia. Similarly, a pure tone hearing screening is performed in the presence of auditory comprehension problem, or auditory agnosia; generally, the recommended protocol for adults over 65 years is screening at the loudness level of 40 decibels for two frequencies (1 and 2 kilohertz).

Occasionally supplementary tests are administered in conjunction with standard language examination. The decision regarding the selection of a supplementary test is made in two possible circumstances: to verify or confirm the identified symptoms; and to reassure that the reported symptoms were not missed during the standard assessment. For example, the *Boston Naming Test* may be administered as a supplementary test for a patient with complaint of anomia, who demonstrated no naming difficulty for standard convergent naming tasks (see Appendix A).

NONSTANDARD ASSESSMENT: LINGUISTIC DESCRIPTION

The term "nonstandard" implies nonadherence to a prescriptive stimulus-response paradigm during assessment. An established nonstandard format for collecting a language sample is the elicitation of connected speech. Typically, an elicited language sample describes the quality and quantity of verbal output and therefore, it is a preferred option for estimating an individual's routine, or functional communication skills. The term *linguistic description,* or conversation analysis, is thus used in any clinical application of this form of assessment protocol. Another rationale for the use of linguistic description in aphasia is to obtain neurolinguistic information, which may be defined as the association between linguistic symptoms and corresponding neurological information that help link language performance to possible etiologies and site of lesion.

Linguistic description aims to determine the type and degree of impairment for the four linguistic parameters including phonology, semantics, morphosyntactics and pragmatics. The first two parameters (phonology and semantics) reflect the integrity in the use of symbols/concepts, while the latter two (morpho-syntactics and pragmatics) represent the use of rules for manipulating the phonological and semantic (or lexical) symbols to convey information.

Procedures for language description first require elicitation of sufficient verbal output (5–10 minutes in length) from the speaker with minimal interjection or intrusion from other communication partner(s). The possibility of obtaining relatively extensive amount of qualitative information with this brief interaction period is an appealing feature of this form of assessment. Some examples for eliciting uninterrupted connected speech include posing open-ended questions seeking information on familiar topics (family, work, medical history or hobby), generating monologues (describing a favorite vacation, movie or town), describing a structured procedure (cook an egg or change a tire), or describe pictures (single or multiple frames) depicting multiple referents and actions (Cherepski & Drummond, 1987; Drummond & Simmons, 1995; Drummond & Boss, 2004). The obtained verbal output can be transcribed to describe/characterize the performance across each of the four linguistic parameters or it can be exposed some rating scale using specified criteria (see Table 7.2). Typically, identification of errors and error patterns are examined to expedite the evaluation procedure and fulfill the need to identify the communication symptoms. It is important to note that not all linguistic parameters may be equally impaired in a given patient. Also, the linguistic context/situation can affect the occurrence of select errors or aphasic symptoms.

Some of the language-specific symptoms defined in Chapter 6 are examined under the four linguistic parameters:

PHONOLOGICAL VARIABLES: Through this linguistic parameter the integrity in accessing and sequencing appropriate phonological symbols for word production is examined; this focus excludes the need for detailed phonetic (sound) description. Typically, any deviation in the production of consonantal or syllable segment in a word is identified as a phonological error. Such errors in word production are thus determined as phonemic (or literal) paraphasia and/or neologistic paraphasia.

MORPHO-SYNTACTIC VARIABLES: The term "morpho" is derived from "morpheme", which represents a minimal grammatical unit (or "function word"). Grammatical morphemes can either independently convey meaning as a single word, also termed "free" morpheme (e.g., "come"); or they may be represented as "bound" morphemes when they occur as prefixes and suffixes in a word (e.g., "_ing" in the word "coming"). The term "syntactical" refers to grammar (or syntax), which implies organization of a series of words to formu-

Table 7.2. A Checklist for Identifying Symptoms for the Four Linguistic Parameters.

Linguistic Parameter and Symptoms	Severity Rating			
	Absent	Occasionally present	Frequently present	Excessive
Phonology				
Phonemic/literal paraphasia (Circle one)	1	2	3	4
Neologistic paraphasia (Circle one)	1	2	3	4
Morphosyntactics				
Verbal Fluency (Circle one)	Fluent	Nonfluent	Mixed	
Agrammatic utterance (Circle one)	1	2	3	4
Paragrammatic utterance (Circle one)	1	2	3	4
Semantics				
Word retrieval problem (Circle one)	1	2	3	4
Types of word retrieval behaviors:				
Hesitation/pausing/interjection (Circle one)	1	2	3	4
Revision/self-correction (Circle one)	1	2	3	4
Repetition (part-/whole word) (Circle one)	1	2	3	4
Verbal/semantic paraphasia (Circle one)	1	2	3	4
Anaphor/indefinite words (Circle one)	1	2	3	4
Circumlocution (Circle one)	1	2	3	4
Pragmatics				
Irrelevancies/noncohesiveness (Circle one)	1	2	3	4
Types of irrelevancies:				
Referencing error (Circle one)	1	2	3	4
Conjoining error (Circle one)	1	2	3	4
Ellipses error (Circle one)	1	2	3	4

late a sentence. Syntactic adequacy can be described as phrase length, number of information units, or sentence accuracy and completeness. Frequently, concepts such as "average phrase length" and "mean length of utterance/response" (MLU/MLR) also refer to syntactic efficiency. Usually MLU/MLR is computed as the ratio of total words divided by total number of utterances/responses in which an utterance is defined through the following verbal behaviors:

- Production of a grammatically complete sentence.
- Discernable drop in inflection, or falling juncture toward the end of a phrase or sentence.
- Obvious and prolong silent periods (or pauses) between consecutive responses.

Such factors, as well as calculation of speaking rate (ratio of speech output time and total speaking time) and other prosodic features (intonation/inflection and pausing) help differentiate nonfluent versus fluent verbal output. Additionally, incomplete and erroneous productions of phrases and utterances are readily identified as either telegrammatism or paragrammatism through language sampling.

SEMANTIC VARIABLES: Semantics is generally discussed as word meaning in neurolinguistic literature. It reflects a clustering of select perceptual features that lead to the creation of a "lexicon" (or word/vocabulary) commonly used by all members within a linguistic society. Each word denotes a specific meaning; for example, "dog" implies a domestic animal with four legs and unique physical characteristics and sound generating pattern). An error, or struggle to retrieve a target word is thus identified as a word retrieval problem (anomia); generally such problems are observed during the production of nouns, verbs, and adjectives. Research findings indicate that frequently used words are easier to retrieve than less frequently used words. Similarly, attributes pertaining to self (personal and animate nouns), operative/manipulative words, word pairs (antonyms), and obvious word functions (agent or object) are relatively easier to retrieve.

The use of semantic paraphasia, circumlocution and anaphor are obvious indicators of a word retrieval problem. The relative occurrences of each of these error manifestations can be observed during connected speech; such productions can also evaluate word retrieval strategies that lead to successful word retrieval of the target word. Some overt signs of struggle toward accessing the lexicon can be reflected through the following verbal behaviors:

- *Hesitations* and *interjections* are obvious silent or verbal pauses preceding the retrieval of target words (e.g., "um . . . table"). This characteristic is prevalent in both brain damaged and nonbrain damaged individuals.
- *Revision,* or self-correction of an incorrect word until there is successful retrieval of the target word is also a sign of search toward lexicon retrieval (e.g., "book. No . . . chair; no . . . table").
- *Part-* or *whole-word repetition* is single or multiple repetitions of the initial syllable (" ta . . . ta . . . table") or the entire target word ("table . . . table; yes, table"). Again, the repetitions reflect covert struggle, postponement to commit to a response, and perhaps verification of the retrieved word.

Although each of the above signs attest to successful access and retrieval of the word from long-term storage, their occurrence in conversation suggest either a phonological struggle with pronouncing the syllables, or that they reflect observable self-monitoring behaviors. Such behaviors are therefore considered as favorable self-cuing strategies; they are generally associated with normal aging and with relatively less severe word retrieval problems.

PRAGMATIC VARIABLES: Pragmatics relates to language use based on established rules within a given culture. The preservation of these rules during verbal output is determined through semantic relevancy (or appropriateness) and "cohesion," which implies that the series of utterances contribute to the continuity and meaning of the conversation topic (or topic-focus organization). Research indicates that a positive relationship exists between increased verbosity (quantity of output) and impaired topic-focus organization/irrelevancy in aphasia (Drummond, 1986). Although some degree of verbal fluency enhances meaningful communication, sometimes the limited verbal output observed in severe aphasia can also serve some pragmatic functions. For example, aphasic individuals whose verbal repertoire is restricted to exclusive use of automatic speech (e.g., "I guess so") have been able to employ them to convey speech acts that require a comment or a response; their automatic utterances have also served as a strategy for revising conversational attempts (McElduff & Drummond, 1991). Additionally, severe aphasic individuals have been observed to utilize nonverbal behaviors such as smiles/laughter to serve pragmatic functions of either protesting or rejecting their conversational partner's verbal output; these individuals also use smiling as a discourse strategy to maintain their presence in a conversation (Norris & Drummond, 1998).

Noncohesive utterances are frequently examined through the occurrence of following errors:

- Referencing error reflects the absence of a referent (topic or subject) in an utterance (e.g., "The only thing is (um) this and that").
- Disagreement between co-referential pronouns can be observed through misuse of either person or number (e.g., "He came to see me and I told her/them I was busy").
- Conjoining error is observed in utterances that link elements through use of conjunctions or relative clauses; the linked elements do not convey an appropriate, or acceptable, meaning

(e.g., "Swim all the way so we weren't much in it").

- Ellipsis, or information, errors are identified if there is deletion or misstatement of the content; the verbal context does not help identify the missing element (e.g., "I worked very hard when I was . . . , and then I had twins").

Although the different linguistic variables are commonly examined in connected speech elicitations, they can also be identified in standard communication assessments. Linguistic symptoms can be substantiated during the assessment of the two primary modalities of auditory comprehension and verbal expression (see Table 7.1). For example, impaired auditory comprehension (listening) and poor self-monitoring can be linked to pragmatic (irrelevant and tangential responses), semantic (word retrieval), morphosyntactic (paragrammatism) and phonological problems.

The four linguistic parameters and symptoms therein, can also be linked to one another. For example, the connection between morphosyntactic and semantic breakdown can be seen through the prevalence of telegrammatism (morphosyntactic problem) and hesitations (semantic problem); the halted, disrupted flow of speech is the linking factor for each of these linguistic symptoms. Correspondingly, paragrammatic utterances (morphosyntactic problem) are associated with increased use of verbal paraphasia, word repetitions and anaphors which define semantic breakdown; these verbal characteristics can also be identified as referencing, ellipsis and conjoining errors within the linguistic parameter of pragmatics.

DIALECTICAL VARIATIONS: A distinction needs to be made between verbal elicitations from individuals who use vernacular, or nonstandard variants of English and aphasic linguistic errors. For example, during phonological description the occurrence of "aks" for "ask" should not be considered a phonemic paraphasia since such phonological substitution tends to occur among some African-American English speakers. Similarly, morphosyntactic variations in nonstandard English should not be identified as paragrammatisms. Some examples of such dialectical variations include the following examples:

- Bound morpheme variations in use of suffixes in verbs ("I does; I goes"), omission of past tense marker ("-ed"), deletion of adverbial marker ("-ly"), deletion of adjectival markers denoting comparatives ("-er") and superlatives ("-est"), omission pronominal

contractions ("he going"), and deletion of plural ("-s") or posses-
sive ("-'s") during noun productions.

- Verb form variations through person-number disagreement ("they was" or "she have"), use of infinitives ("he be going"), or deletion of auxiliary verb ("he going").
- Variations in modifiers such as substitution of indefinites ("a" for "an").
- Variations in question formation through deletion of preposing auxiliary verb (" you going?" for "are you going?") or inversion of question form ("You are going?").
- Variations in the use of negations ("ain't" for "am not") or use of double negatives ("I know no nobody").

ASSESSMENT OF COGNITIVE-COMMUNICATION

Cognition is an umbrella term that includes a variety of low (simple) and high (complex) order functions of the brain. An impairment of even few of its myriad components can adversely affect communication and, therefore, cognitive functions are evaluated either preceding or concurrent with standard language assessment. The components of cognitive assessment include the following areas:

- *Arousal/consciousness* and *attention* involve observation of behavioral responses to any form of external verbal (call the patient by name), tactile (touch or move an arm), visual (direct light to the patient's face) or thermal (touch face with a cold object) stimuli. A lack of an overt response is reflective of disturbance in consciousness or evidence of coma; it is generally associated with extensive brain damage and is considered as a predictor of adverse outcome. Attention may be evaluated through the ability to maintain focus, or resist distraction, while engaged in an informal conversation, or during a structured activity (match pictures). Although a 20-minute attention to a structured task or activity is considered "normal," the duration of attention is strongly influenced by intrinsic (physiological status, fatigue, or preference/interest) and extrinsic factors (communication partner, topic, or time of day).
- *Affective behaviors* and *reactions* during communicative interactions are assessed to gauge their appropriateness. Any evidence of euphoria, increased egocentricity, emotional lability, excessive

and inappropriate use of affective language, or catastrophic reactions is noted to estimate the impact of each of these behaviors on communication competency.

- *Perceptual problems* are generally reflected through the presence of visual and/or auditory agnosias. Visual agnosias are assessed through tasks that require visual scanning/tracking, visual matching/discrimination and visual-spatial processing. Auditory agnosias may be assessed through matching tones representing different frequencies and loudness, discriminating nonspeech and speech sounds, as well as word recognitions.

- *Orientation to person, space and time* is evaluated by seeking answers to questions pertaining to personal/biographical information (e.g., name), immediate physical environment (e.g., institution, city or state), and temporal events (e.g., days of week or season).

- *Amnesia:* Memories are generally created when nerve cells in a circuit increase the strength of their connections (synapses) and they are stored in two storage systems: *short-term* (STM) and *long-term memory* (LTM). New, or moment-to-moment, information is typically held in temporary storage, or STM. This is possible due to a temporary strengthening of the synapse whose effect can last for several minutes to hours. The amount of information that can be stored in STM is limited to seven items (plus or minus 2 items); this ability can be assessed through the recall of a string of words or numbers. If the information is considered as important for permanent storage, then it is placed in LTM. This process of consolidating information requires a chain of events involving release of special synapse-strengthening proteins that result in repeated stimulation of select circuits (LTP) to ultimately result in permanent storage. Figure 7.1 provides a hierarchical organization of the different components of LTM. Information from LTM can be accessed or retrieved with the help of internal or external cues and are therefore assigned to two distinct categories: Implicit and explicit memories. Long-term *implicit memory* is further organized as procedural and emotional memories. *Procedural memory* involves routine, long-remembered skills such as brushing one's teeth. *Emotional memories* are created by the interactions between the amygdala, hippocampus, prefrontal cortex and the autonomic nervous system. For example, the amygdala perceives a threatening stimulus/situation, the prefrontal cortex assesses the situation and makes a judgment, the sympathetic division of the autonomic nervous system secretes epinephrine to increase the heart and respiratory rate and sharpens the senses, and the hippocampus stores this experience as STM and LTM. Long-term *explicit memory* is further arranged as semantic, episodic and iconic memories. *Semantic memory* relates to recall of factual information (e.g., sour grape); *episodic,* or *event-related, memory* pertains to recall of previous personal experiences (e.g., birthday celebration or favorite vacation). The third category, *iconic memory,* involves the recall of information that relies primarily on visual symbols (e.g., traffic signs). Breakdown in each, or any of these memories may be deemed as *retrograde amnesia,* which is defined as the impaired recall of recent or LTM. Sometimes the term *anterograde amnesia* is used to characterize the impaired ability to learn/retain new information or recall it from STM; it can be assessed via recalling a specific word at different stages of the examination. Recent literature on "false memories" poses questions regarding the objectivity of assessing emotional and episodic memories because their accuracies tend to be influenced by factors such as imagination and honesty.

- The communication components of any cognitive assessment include the two primary language modalities of *auditory comprehension* (e.g., simple and complex information/commands) and *verbal expression* (divergent and convergent word retrieval, verbal fluency, and linguistic relevancy). The different subtests within each of these two modalities are thus included in any cognitive-communication assessment.

- *Abstract reasoning* or *executive functions* are evaluated through several types of tasks: problem solving (e.g., logical deduction), sequencing of information (e.g., delineating steps for accomplishing a task), calculation (e.g., money management or simple arithmetic), planning and execution (goal formulation, scheduling and accomplishing tasks, or seeking alternative actions/options), and interpretation of metaphoric language (idioms, metaphors and proverbs).

It is important to note that each of the different cognitive functions serves as pre- or co-requisites for successful communication and therefore, they are generally included in standard communication/language assessment (see Table 7.1). Examples of standard tests for assessing

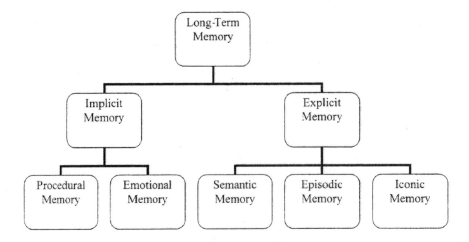

Figure 7.1. Different types of long-term memories.

overall mental and cognitive-communication functions are also included in the Appendix A.

Finally, a distinction needs to be made between cognitive decline and cognitive impairment. A decline in cognitive-communication implies a gradual regression of once normal functions as implicated in the progressive changes in brain and behavior associated with dementia. In contrast, cognitive-communication impairment characterizes those impairments resulting from sudden onset nonprogressive brain lesions associated with TBI and right (nondominant) hemisphere CVAs.

ASSESSMENT OF FUNCTIONAL COMMUNICATION

Functional communication relates to a person's ability to interact with others in routine, daily situations either within the context of the family, friends or strangers. It can reflect an integration of the different components of linguistic and cognitive processes that are generally evaluated through formal assessment protocols. Therefore, assessment of functional communication can observe a range of physical, mental, communicative (or social) functions; it is applicable to individuals who have sustained a CVA, dementia or TBI. Its rationale is trifold: diagnose the presence of a disorder, determine eligibility for rehabilitation, and reduce the cost for service delivery. This form of assessment has the potential to provide information regarding the individual's optimal ability to communicate at school or work, and in general social interactions; sometimes it is also referred as a determiner of functional "outcome."

As a general rule, functional communication assessment protocols tend to be expedient and relatively flexible in their administration; the patient may not even be aware of undergoing an assessment. Such measures tend to utilize rating scales to report clinical observations; related information may be collected by any member of the multidisciplinary team (nursing, occupational therapy and speech-language pathology), and it may be obtained at patient admission and/or discharge. Although the obtained data provide quantitative information, they do reflect subjective impressions regarding the patient's interaction ability. It also needs to be cautioned that no functional outcome scale is appropriate for every clinical population. However, this form of assessment is federally endorsed via organizations such as the National Institutes of Health (NIH), managed care organizations (MCOS) and health maintenance organizations (HMOs). The advantages of using functional communication measures are their time and cost effectiveness, and their potential for determining treatment effectiveness and efficiency. Paradoxically, their use may foster apprehension regarding elimination of services or shorten the length of treatment for patients and thus lead to ethical concerns relating to documentation of false positive outcome to justify continuation of treatment services to patients.

Functional communication assessment protocols evaluate cognitive and social communication skills. Related procedures assess cognitive-communication competency through an estimation of attention, memory, and executive functions; social aspects of communication are evaluated through the inference of pragmatic skills, social behaviors, and need or opportunities for communication. An example of a related protocol is the *Functional Communication Measures* (FCM) available through the *American Speech-Language Association* (Frattali, Thompson, Holland, Wohl & Ferketic, 1995). The FCM utilizes a seven-point scale to measure outcomes in 12 areas pertaining to language (comprehension and production of spoken, written and nonverbal language), cognitive-communication, swallowing, speech (voice and fluency), and hearing. A popular option, the *Ranchos Los Amigos* (RLA) *Levels of Cognitive Functions* estimates the degree of communicative independence by utilizing a severity-based model, which assigns an individual to one of eight possible levels where Level I implies "no response" (or very severe) and Level VIII reflects "purposeful and appropriate" behavior (Hagen, Malkmus & Durham, 1979). Recently the *Functional Communication Scale* (FCS) evaluates the adequacy of 12 communication items (speech intelligibility, speech rhythm and intonation, word usage, grammar usage, revision, relevancy, verbosity, turn-taking, topic initiation, topic maintenance, emotional stability, and attention) though use of a three-point rating scale (Drummond & Boss, 2004). Sections of other measures also estimate communication performance of individuals with brain damage. One such measure is the *Functional Independence Measure* (FIM) which estimates 18 functions utilizing a seven-point rating scale. A problem with the FIM is that only five of its 18 items directly address communication and related cognitive functions (Research Foundation, 1990).

SUMMARY

The outcome of any viable assessment protocol should yield information regarding the severity of the aphasia; this is generally inferred from the elicited scores four each modality and across the four modalities. During such interpretation it is important to consider that the four language modalities are interdependent; the two comprehension modalities augment each other, and they in turn influence the preferred (or residual) expression modalities. One cannot presume that the degree of impairment is "flat" (or similar) across all four modalities; each patient has some residual strengths and weaknesses and the fundamental clinical objective should be to identify them. Previous research indicates that all aphasic individuals demonstrate some degree of comprehension (auditory and/visual) problem, and the magnitude of impairment in these two modalities typically contributes to the severity of the aphasia. The other equally important focus during interpretation of test performance is to determine the type (or classification) of aphasia and cognitive-communication problem, as well as highlight the corresponding symptoms. This goal also considers qualitative factors such as the effect of stimulus/task, type and frequency of errors.

The clinical assessment protocol summarizes information from all sources including the background history, results of structured modality-based tests, informal language and behavioral-cognitive performances, and other special tests. A typical diagnostic report begins with a summary of personal information regarding the patient's age, medical history including etiology and diagnosis, localization information, date of onset, concurrent health problems, and education and occupation. The test findings are highlighted through the provision of scores for the four language modalities and related tasks within each. Greater attention is given to the observed performances for the two primary modalities: auditory comprehension and verbal expression. This is reflected in distinguishing the influence of perceptual and cognitive factors on language comprehension and production. Elicited connected speech should identify the linguistic parameter(s) that is the most and least impaired, and determines the type of verbal fluency with primary verbal characteristics. The observed verbal characteristics should relate to possible clinical communication symptoms as well. The need for any modification to the testing protocol including any variables that facilitated or exacerbated the language symptoms should be documented in the assessment report. Also, the potential impact of the aphasia, or the cognitive-communication problem and related symptoms, on the patient's ability to perform routine daily activities should be briefly explained. Finally, the prognosis for recovery, or possible outcome, should be speculated based on highlighting some favorable factors from the background information and test findings. It needs to be noted that the length of an assessment report is dictated by the targeted reader, i.e., a professional peer, another health care provider, the patient's employer, or the reimbursement agency.

Determination of "normalcy" needs to be carefully considered because it does foster clinical dilemma. Sometimes this reference is used to infer adequacy for routine communication but at other times seeks optimal performance. For example, if successfully completing two-step commands is the standard observation among nonbrain damaged adults, then why do the auditory comprehension subtests of standard tests require completion of three-step commands? Correspondingly, verbal output of nonbrain damaged adults is rich in syntactical and semantic deviations as reflected through interjections, automatisms and fragmented utterances; the same linguistic observations are considered "abnormal" simply because the individual has a positive history of brain damage.

Appendix A

A LIST OF SOME STANDARD LANGUAGE AND COGNITIVE COMMUNICATION ASSESSMENT PROTOCOLS

Title	Authors
Language Screening Tests	
Aphasia Language Performance Scale	Keenan, J., and Brassell, E. (1975)
Sklar Aphasia Scale	Sklar, M. (1973)
Bedside Evaluation Screening Test for Aphasia	Sand, E., and Fitch-West, J. (1987)
Comprehensive Language Tests	
Boston Diagnostic Aphasia Examination	Goodglass, H. Kaplan, E., and Barressi, B. (2000)
Communicative Abilities in Daily Living	Holland, A. (1980)
Western Aphasia Battery	Kertesz, A. (1982)
Porch Index of Communicative Ability	Porch, B. (1981)
Cognitive Communication Screening Tests	
Glascow Coma Scale	Teasdale, G., and Jennett, B. (1974)
Mini Mental State Examination	Folstein, M., Folstein, S., and McHugh, P. (1975)
Comprehensive Cognitive-Communication Tests	
Galveston Orientation & Amnesia Test	Levin, H., O'Donnell, V., and Grossman, R. (1979)
Ross Information Processing Ability	Ross-Swain, D (1996)
Arizona Battery for Communication Disorders of Dementia	Bayles, K., and Tomoeda, C. (1991)
Supplementary Tests	
Auditory Comprehension Test for Sentences	Shewan, C. (1978)
Revised Token Test	McNeil, M., and Prescott, T. (1978)
Reading Comprehension Battery	LaPointe L., and Horner, J. (1979)
Apraxia Battery for Adults	Dabul, B. (2000)
Boston Naming Test	Kaplan, E., Goodglass, H., and Weintraub, S. (2001)

Title	Authors
Mini Inventory of Right Brain Injury	Pimental, P., and Kingsbury, N. (1989)
Raven's Coloured Progressive Matrices	Raven, J. (1995)
Visual Retention Test	Benton, A. (1992)
Visual Organization Test	Hooper, H. (1983)
Wisconsin Card Sorting Test	Grant, D., and Berg, E. (1993)
Functional Communication Assessments	
Ranchos Los Amigos Scale	Hagen, C, Malkmus, D., and Durham, P. (1979)
Functional Communication Scale	Drummond, S., and Boss, M. (2004)
Functional Independence Measures	Research Foundation (1990)
Functional Communication Measures	Frattali, C. (1995)

Appendix B

SAMPLE LANGUAGE SCREENING FORMAT

Patient Name: _____ Age/Date of Birth: _____ Test Date: _____

Medical Date:_____

Scoring: 0=Incorrect/No response; 1=Assisted correct response; 2=Partially correct/distorted response; 3=Delayed correct response; 4=Correct response

Modality and Tasks	Stimulus Items	Scoring	Comment
I. Auditory Comprehension			
Object identification (Recognition) Single(simple) commands	1. Point to the telephone 2. Point to the pen 3. Point to what is (color). 4. Point to what is (shape).	0 1 2 3 4 0 1 2 3 4 0 1 2 3 4 0 1 2 3 4	
Answer 'Yes-No' questions/ Orientation	1. Is your name (wrong name)? 2. Does it snow in July? 3. Do you live in ____? 4. Can a horse fly?	0 1 2 3 4 0 1 2 3 4 0 1 2 3 4 0 1 2 3 4	
Axial commands	1. Make a fist. 2. Close your eyes. 3. Point to your left ear. 4. Touch your right arm.	0 1 2 3 4 0 1 2 3 4 0 1 2 3 4 0 1 2 3 4	
Multiple (complex) commands	1. Look at the clock & turn on the TV. 2. Pick up the pen & keys & give them to me. 3. Put the pen and keys next to the paper. 4. Pick up the paper, no, just the keys.	0 1 2 3 4 0 1 2 3 4 0 1 2 3 4 0 1 2 3 4	

Continued

II. Verbal Expression			
Object naming (convergent retrieval)	1. What is this? (point to a cup)	0 1 2 3 4	
	2. What is this? (point to the pen)	0 1 2 3 4	
	3. What is this? (point to the window)	0 1 2 3 4	
	4. What is this? (point to the light/lamp)	0 1 2 3 4	
Sentence completion (convergent retrieval)	1. The grass is —-? (green)	0 1 2 3 4	
	2. Sugar is —-? (sweet)	0 1 2 3 4	
	3. You can write with a —? (pen/pencil)	0 1 2 3 4	
	4. We go to the restaurant to —? (eat)	0 1 2 3 4	
Automatic (rote) sequencing	1. Count from 1 to 20 (let's begin with 1–).	0 1 2 3 4	
	2. Name the days of the week (start with Sunday–).	0 1 2 3 4	
Word and sentence repetition	1. Say the word - Bed.	0 1 2 3 4	
	2. Say the word - Pencil.	0 1 2 3 4	
	3. The window is open.	0 1 2 3 4	
	4. The girl & boy are playing.	0 1 2 3 4	
Connected speech	Elicit spontaneous verbal output using familiar topic(s) to code for the following: Fluent (F) or Nonfluent (NF) Telegrammatism (T), Paragrammatism (P) or Normal Verbal Irrelevancy Jargon: Semantic (S) or Neologistic (N) or NA	F NF T P N 0 1 2 3 4 S N NA	
III. Reading Comprehension			
Word and picture identification	1. Match letters represented as upper and lower cases.	0 1 2 3 4	
	2. Match words represented in print and script forms.	0 1 2 3 4	
	3. Match coins (dimes/nickels/ quarter)	0 1 2 3 4	
	4. Match objects by colors (red/ green/yellow)	0 1 2 3 4	

Continued

Sentence comprehension (Respond to instructions written in lower case)	1. Pick up the pen.	0 1 2 3 4	
	2. Circle words with the letter 'R'.	0 1 2 3 4	
	3. Point to the window.	0 1 2 3 4	
	4. Point to your left ear.	0 1 2 3 4	
IV. Written Expression			
Copying: words and sentence	1. Pen	0 1 2 3 4	
	2. Window	0 1 2 3 4	
	3. Numbers 1–10	0 1 2 3 4	
	4. It is time to take a nap.	0 1 2 3 4	
Spontaneous output	1. Write your full name.	0 1 2 3 4	
	2. Write your home address.	0 1 2 3 4	
Total Score and Severity	Mild=141–180; Moderate=101–140; Severe=61–100; Profound=below 60	/180	

Check (√) all that apply: Hemiplegia/Hemiparesis __; Dysarthria __; Apraxia __; Visual/Auditory Agnosia __; Attention/Cognitive Problems __

Chapter 8

CLASSIFICATION AND DIFFERENTIAL DIAGNOSIS

Differences among normal individuals are an acceptable fact and so are differences between individuals with brain damage. The presentation of clusters of clinical symptoms has led to segregating these individuals into select groups, or *classification categories.* One of the rationale for administering a battery of assessment tasks is to derive at a classification through the process of *differential diagnosis,* which involves an ongoing review of observed symptoms in the context of available medical and personal history. The basis for classification is to associate a cluster of characteristics (symptoms) to a communication disorder; this practice facilitates sharing of clinical information among the involved professions. The fundamental objective of any classification system is to promote optimal patient intervention and recovery, and direct the clinician to select appropriate treatment options and strategies for the prevailing symptoms.

Classifications incorporate neurological information relating to site of lesion (anterior/prerolandic versus posterior/postrolandic, or right versus left hemisphere) or nature of lesion (progressive versus non-progressive, ischemic versus traumatic). They also encompass cognitive-communication information regarding residual comprehension and production proficiency, or perceptual and cognitive problems; and they integrate linguistic information pertaining to verbal fluency (nonfluent versus fluent) and verbal insufficiencies (paraphasias, irrelevancies, or telegrammatism and paragrammatism). Although each classification category represents a unique cluster of symptoms, it may also include generic symptoms such as apraxia, anomia, amnesia, or agnosia. This chapter describes the classification categories for aphasias and cognitive-communication disorders. Also highlighted is the relationship between aphasia and premorbid communication related issues, and draws attention to factors that can help distinguish between the different types of communication disorders. The final section pertains to the delineation of key prognostic variables that can be used as guidance for determining rehabilitation potential.

APHASIA CLASSIFICATION

A couple of clinical features commonly characterize all aphasic individuals and they include damage to the language-dominant hemisphere and the presence of word retrieval problems (or anomia). Thereafter, there is sufficient evidence to group aphasic individuals according to esoteric collection of prevailing symptoms to best describe their language disorder. Confirmed documentation of collection of symptoms, with supportive neuropathological evidence, has led to current classification for aphasia.

Historically, aphasia classification originated from the concepts of *sensory versus motor* dichotomy introduced by neurologists such as Carl Wernicke during the nineteenth century. This neurological perspective shifted to the psychological notion of *receptive* versus *expressive aphasia.* Each of these binary systems has been deemed inadequate because aphasic individuals tend to manifest concomitant features reflecting both receptive (sensory) and expressive (motor) deficits. Based on these clinical observations, a variety of four-category classifications were introduced in the first half of the twentieth century. For example, the psychological parameters of language modalities (listening, speaking, reading and writing), introduced between the 1930s through the 1950s, were rapidly adapted in aphasia assessment and classification. Gradually, clinical practice mandated integration of test results, observation of linguistic verbal behaviors, and available neurological information on lesion localization as essential ingredients for aphasia classification. Contemporary classifications therefore, reflect these contributions to help delineate a composite of symptoms/features for each major category each of which is summarized in Table 8.1, and also described in this section.

- *Global Aphasia:* This category is assigned to the most severe type

Table 8.1. Typical Classification Categories for Aphasia.

Type	Site of Lesion	Comprehension	Spontaneous speech	Repetition
Global	Extensive left. hemispheric/ perisylvian; fronto-temporo-parietal; main trunk of middle cerebral artery involvement	Impaired	Nonfluent (stereotype)	Impaired
Broca's	Frontal/prerolandic/anterior; Broca's and adjacent areas	Relatively preserved	Nonfluent (telegrammatism; apraxia)	Impaired
Transcortical motor (Anterior isolation syndrome)	Deep frontal; white matter; peripheral to Broca's area; beyond perisylvian region; supplementary motor area; association tracts; anterior cerebral artery involvement	Relatively preserved	Nonfluent (echolalia)	Relatively preserved
Jargon	Variable or nonspecific, but large lesion	May/not impaired	Fluent	Impaired
Wernicke's	Temporal/postrolandic/posterior; Wernicke's area; supplemental sensory area	Impaired (word deafness)	Fluent (paragrammatism)	Impaired
Transcortical sensory	Deep temporal; white matter peripheral to Wernicke's area; beyond perisylvian region	Impaired	Fluent (echolalia)	Relatively preserved
Conduction	White matter/deep perisylvian extending to Insula; arcuate fasciculus; nonspecific; auditory association areas involved (T2)	Relatively preserved	Fluent or mixed	Impaired
Anomic	Little anatomic specificity; cortical (angular, supra-marginal); subcortical (thalamic; corpus striatum); small size	Preserved	Fluent	May/not impaired

of aphasia. Individuals representing this group tend to have extensive lesions involving the entire perisylvian region including the surface gray and/or deep tissues that are heavily reliant on the middle cerebral artery. The primary clinical features include moderate to severe comprehension (auditory and visual) problems, and severely reduced expressive (verbal and written) skills. Volitional/spontaneous verbal output is practically absent and if possible, it may be limited to automatic phrases and verbal stereotypes. Individuals with less extensive lesions may manifest transient symptoms of global aphasia in the early days following the onset of the damage. Such individuals may recover from the severe comprehension deficits and practically absent expressive language to nonfluent-like verbal output and some restoration of comprehension skills if there is preponderance of anterior/pre-rolandic lesion; or their performance may transform to relatively fluent verbal output with persistent comprehension problems if there is a relatively extensive temporo-parietal (posterior) lesion.

- *Broca's Aphasia:* Individuals representing this type of aphasia generally incur a lesion in the frontal lobe of the language-dominant hemisphere involving the Broca's area (or area 44) and adjacent areas. This category is thus associated with suprasylvian, pre-rolandic lesions with, or without, concurrent damage to the deeper white matter. Limited verbal expression is the primary problem in Broca's aphasia when compared to the relatively preserved comprehension skills of these individuals. Linguistically, their verbal output is nonfluent and highlighted by the presence of phonemic paraphasias and agrammatic/telegrammatic utterances. It needs to be noted that such verbal output problems impede the ability of these individuals to repeat words or sentences. Although they may have little or no difficulty with simple/routine auditory comprehension tasks, there may be a breakdown when required to comprehend grammatically complex instructions or materials. Because of the involvement of the frontal lobe these individuals may demonstrate concurrent motor programming difficulties observed as oral and or verbal apraxia, and perhaps limb apraxia. The impaired frontal lobe may also result in contralateral hemiparesis or hemiplegia, which may explain the presence of concurrent dysarthria in this group of individuals.

- *Wernicke's Aphasia:* This classification category is commonly associated with postrolandic lesions involving the cortical areas that receive blood flow via the posterior branches of the middle cerebral artery. The dominant hemisphere's temporal lobe, particularly the posterior superior temporal gyrus or Wernicke's area (areas 21 and 22), is generally compromised. The lesion may also extend to adjacent areas including the middle temporal (T2)and inferior parietal gyri, as well as the angular gyrus and the proximal white matter. Individuals with Wernicke's aphasia have obvious auditory comprehension problems due to the involvement of the temporal lobe, and severe cases are sometimes identified as having word deafness/auditory verbal agnosia. The verbal output of these individuals is fluent with evidence of a variety of paraphasias, presence of paragrammatisms, and conjoining or ellipses errors due to their defective ability to monitor and self-correct erroneous verbal productions.

- *Conduction Aphasia:* This category reflects disordered reproduction of verbal language, which perhaps explains the obvious deficit in repeating auditory-verbal stimuli from STM. The site of lesion for this type of aphasia is associated with medial, white matter lesions extending deep to the insula or the limbic lobe of the language dominant hemisphere. These individuals may also have left hemispheric perisylvian lesions involving the auditory association area (T2), the arcuate fasciculus and/or the supramarginal gyrus. The proximity of these structures to the insula/limbic lobe accounts for their auditory-verbal STM problems; such deficits are frequently identified through impaired verbal (word and sentence) repetition performances. These individuals may demonstrate relatively preserved auditory comprehension for routine communication, but their STM limitations may impede comprehension of longer and complex sentence structures (relative clauses, passives, or determining syntactic relations between lexical items). Verbally, their output is fluent or may be mixed in fluency with paragrammatisms and word retrieval problems; although paraphasias are evident, no one type may predominate. A noteworthy characteristic of conduction aphasia is the relatively better performance on reading and writing modalities than for auditory-verbal tasks; for example, visual repetition of words and sentences may be easier than auditory repetition of the same stimuli.

- *Anomic Aphasia:* This classification category represents the mildest form of aphasia. Auditory and visual comprehension is fairly preserved among these individuals, and their verbal output is fluent with no obvious grammatical problems. The predominant symptom is anomia, or word-finding difficulty, which may be observed through frequent breakdowns in lexicon retrieval that is manifested through a variety of word retrieval behaviors. The site of lesion for this group may be cortical or subcortical in nature. In case of cortical lesion, there may be either little anatomic specificity relative to locus of impairment (frontal, temporal or parietal lobe), or the lesion may be specific to the temporo-parietal (angular and supramarginal gyri) region. Whenever anomic aphasia is determined in the presence of a subcortical lesion, it is generally associated with involvement of either the thalamus or the corpus striatum.

- *Jargon Aphasia:* Occasionally, an individual may be assigned to this classification due to the combination of two factors: predominant use of neologistic jargon in verbal output, and test performance not conforming to any other aphasic type. The site of lesion is the language-dominant hemisphere, and it may extensively involve either the pre- or postrolandic regions. Comprehension may be relatively preserved in the preponderance of a pre-rolandic lesion, but it may be impaired if there is a postrolandic lesion. The presence of undifferentiated neologisms with occasional meaningful words or sterotypes severely disrupts the meaningfulness of verbal output and communication.

- *Transcortical Aphasia:* The term "transcortical," coined by Goldstein (1948), refers to tracts for association processes between various motor and sensory areas. This category is also known as *Isolation Syndrome* implying that the primary language (Wernicke's and Broca's) areas are generally spared while the interconnecting white matter (association tracts) is impaired. The clinical implication for this category is to suggest that the delineated aphasic symptoms are "transient," and that the individual may progress to one of the other aphasic categories over time. Two subtypes of transcortical aphasias are described in the literature one of which is *Transcortical sensory aphasia,* or *Posterior Isolation Syndrome.* This type is characterized by poor comprehension ability, echolalic and fluent verbal output, relatively preserved repetition ability, and difficulty initiating volitional verbal output. The language impairment is due to dissociation of auditory speech area from other language processing areas. The lesion site tends to involve deep posterior parietal or occipito-temporal region. The second subdivision, *Transcortical Motor Aphasia,* or *Anterior Isolation Syndrome,* is characterized by relatively intact auditory comprehension, preserved repetition ability for short phrases, echolalic and yet nonfluent-like verbal output. The site of lesion is white matter that is medial to Broca's area, and tends to be associated with the anterior cerebral artery distribution areas (or parasagittal region).

An important feature of any classification is to recognize that it is "dynamic" in nature, which implies that such categorical assignments are not a permanent reality. It also emphasizes the fact that individuals assigned to one category will (and should) progress to another classification over a period of time to reflect either recovery or decline in functions. Fortunately, individuals who incurred aphasia from nonprogressive brain damage tend to show a pattern of recovery that corresponds to positive shifts in their classification assignments. For example, a patient with the diagnosis of global aphasia may gradually recover to manifest characteristics of Broca's aphasia and then to conduction aphasia. Similarly, an individual with transcortical motor aphasia may also evolve to Broca's aphasia and then to conduction aphasia and ultimately to anomic aphasia. In each of these instances, the patient shifts from a relatively severe disorder to a milder severity representing fewer symptoms; however, each of these transitions maintains/shares verbal nonfluency as a common feature. Correspondingly, patients with fluent verbal output may progress from a severe classification assignment, such as Wernicke's aphasia or transcortical sensory aphasia, to conduction aphasia and finally to anomic aphasia. The only uncanny category is jargon aphasia, which may transcend to either Broca's or Wernicke's aphasia dependent upon the improvement, or nonimprovement, in auditory comprehension. Figure 8.1 depicts the possible directional shifts toward the less severe classification categories.

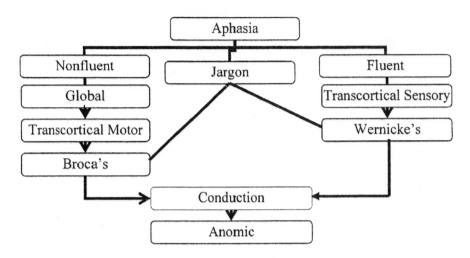

Figure 8.1. Directional shifts in aphasia classification assignments.

ATYPICAL TYPES OF APHASIC DISORDERS

Sometimes an individual may not present the cluster of symptoms that readily conform to one of the common aphasic classification categories. In such instances there may a predominance of one or two symptoms that characterize the language disorder; also, the observed symptoms may be modality-specific. For example, the individual may have obvious manifestations of *pure word deafness* or *auditory verbal agnosia,* where the extensive auditory perceptual problems camouflage the possibility of detecting the clinical symptoms that would otherwise have been designated to the typical Wernicke's aphasia. Another atypical aphasia is *Gerstmann's syndrome,* which is determined in the collective occurrence of the following symptoms: acalculia, finger agnosia, right versus left disorientation, and agraphia. Gerstmann's syndrome is associated with bilateral or unilateral right hemispheric lesion, and it may involve the occipital lobe including the angular gyrus region. Sometimes an individual may acquire exclusive symptoms of *dyslexia with dysgraphia* associated with angular gyrus lesions. Finally, there may be acquired *dyslexia without dysgraphia* (or *pure word blindness*) in lesions exclusive to the visual cortex.

The lesion site may serve as an important consideration for determining atypical aphasia because the observed symptoms do not strictly conform to the expected cortical lesion site(s). This is particularly true with subcortical lesions or lesions involving medial, cortical and subcortical white matter (or "disconnection syndrome"). For example, a subcortical lesion involving the anterior corpus striatum (basal ganglia and the internal capsule) may result in nonfluent aphasic-like symptoms that may not be clearly distinguishable as Broca's aphasia; correspondingly, posterior striatal lesions may result in fluent aphasic-like problems that do not clearly resemble Wernicke's aphasia. In each of these subcortical lesions, there is disruption of the connections between the corpus striatum and the frontal and temporal lobes, respectively. Extensive lesions of corpus striatum may also present with global aphasic-like behaviors, and sometimes dysarthria may occur as a concurrent problem among individuals with subcortical aphasia. Another subcortical site is thalamic lesion where the individual may demonstrate symptoms of anomic aphasia or mild cognitive-communication disorder, characterized by memory and verbal abstraction problems. Such problems have also been observed in nearly one-half of the individuals who have undergone ventrolateral thalamotomy for management of movement disorders (Alarie-Bibeau & Andrianopoulos, 2003). Finally, *crossed aphasia* is determined when the damaged hemisphere and the preferred hand share the same side, or there is an ipsilateral relationship between handedness and site of lesion (left-handers with left hemisphere damage); otherwise, individuals with crossed aphasia may show linguistic symptoms that can be readily assigned to any of the conventional types of aphasia.

APHASIA AND PRE-EXISTING FORMS OF COMMUNICATION

The traditional concept of aphasia has been based on the premise that aphasia is a reflection of an impaired auditory-verbal communication. As such, corresponding symptoms and classifications have been derived from contributions from traditional psychological, neurological and linguistic theories that focus on the quality and quantity of verbal output. This viewpoint has been broadened in the latter part of the twentieth century to include other groups of linguistic communities.

One unique group is deaf individuals who use sign language for communication. Neuroanatomical evidence shows differences between congenitally deaf and normal hearing individuals in regard to the white matter involving the Heschl's gyrus and the temporal lobe. Deaf individuals have been observed to have significantly lower proportion of white matter, which is attributed to the need for fewer connections within the auditory cortex due to their hearing loss (Allen et al., 2004). Functionally, normal elderly deaf individuals who are lifelong users of *American Sign Language* (ASL) show *sign finding problems* that is analogous to the declining word finding ability among normal elderly speech users. This similarity between sign and verbal language users is shared in the presence of a brain damage as well. For example, symptoms resulting from right (nondominant) hemisphere damage tend to be similar in deaf sign users and nonsign users; both hearing and nonhearing individuals demonstrate poor performance on visual-spatial tasks and show neglect for their left side. Similarly, both signers and nonsigners acquire aphasic symptoms subsequent to a left hemisphere lesion; this clinical occurrence provides further evidence for localization of language functions in the left hemisphere irrespective of the presence or absence of a congenital hearing loss. Deaf signers with aphasia also demonstrate performances that conform to the typical types of aphasia (e.g., nonfluent versus fluent; Brocas' versus Wernicke's). Each of these observations de-mystify the contention that since hand gestures used for sign language rely on visual-spatial perception and production, this unique ability should be impaired following a right hemisphere lesion. Thus, it appears that neural organization for sign and verbal language is indistinguishable at the cortical level, and that left hemisphere dominance for language function is not solely dependent on life-long use of the primary sensory (auditory and visual) processes (Bellugi, Poizner & Klima, 1983).

Individuals from diverse linguistic and cultural (ethnicity and geography) backgrounds, particularly nonstandard English speakers, represent another subgroup of interest. Although there is sufficient information attesting that these groups of individuals use nonstandard forms of verbal productions that are observed as phonological, morpho-syntactic and semantic variations, related information on them when they acquire aphasia is strictly anecdotal in nature. The limited information on individuals who use more than one (*bilingual*) or multiple (*polyglot*) languages indicates that when these individuals acquire aphasia, they conform to the principles of *linguistic universals* which implies that their clinical symptoms (such as anomia, paragrammatism, paraphasia) in one language tend to prevail in the other language(s) in their repertoire. However, bilinguals (and polyglots) also demonstrate variability in the relative severity of the observed symptoms for the different languages. Generally, these individuals begin to use the language that is most frequently used at the time of onset of the aphasia. It is also observed that a bilingual or polyglot aphasic individual will maintain the premorbid language switching behavior when interacting with speakers/listeners of different languages. Similarly, these individuals may employ their different languages for selective purposes; for example, they may use one language when expressing emotions (or *affectional language*) and use another when communicating in formal situations. Regarding trend in recovery, it appears that there is a greater recovery for the most frequently used language; also, a reciprocal relationship exists between affectional (emotional) and functional language implying that the affectional language recedes as functional language improves in these individuals (Albert et al., 1981; Minkowski, 1963).

CLASSIFICATION OF
COGNITIVE-COMMUNICATION DISORDERS

A common characteristic of all types of cognitive-communication disorders is that each of these disorders represents a unique neuropathology. Categorization of cognitive-communication disorders is difficult because these disorders result from a conglomeration of neurological diagnoses which themselves have their own esoteric classifications. Two common examples include traumatic brain injury and right hemisphere injury. Other disorders are clustered according to their foremost cognitive symptoms of which two major categories serve as representatives of the myriad possibilities: language of confusion and dementia. This section has therefore described each of these four prominent classification groups that are typically associated with cognitive-communication disorders.

Traumatic Brain Injury (TBI)

Head injuries are classified in different ways. The most common classification dichotomizes open versus closed head injuries. *Open head injury* (OHI) is an observable penetrating sign on the scalp, skull or meninges that indicates that the individual has been a victim of a trauma to the head. Some examples of OHI are gunshot wound, skull fracture, or a laceration. In contrast, a *closed head injury* (CHI) documents the traumatic event even through there is no overt sign of a head injury; there is jarring of the neural tissue from the abrupt changes in mechanical forces involving the contact and inertia. The victim may report a concussion or a contusion to the head, which may have resulted in an epidural, subdural, or subarachnoid hematoma. Another classification system focuses on the site of damage through use of terms such as coup, contrecoup, or coup-contrecoup injury. A *coup injury* is the damage to brain at the site of impact, while *contrecoup injury* implies that the side opposite to the impacted side has suffered the damage (see Figure 5.2, p. 81). Finally, *coup-contrecoup injury* indicates that both, the impacted and opposite side, are damaged.

Individuals with TBI may manifest clusters of symptoms that may conform to the aphasia classifications, and sometimes this unique etiologic group may present combinations of speech-language and perceptual-cognitive symptoms that justify their discussion as an esoteric cognitive-communication disorder. Sometimes however, during the acute or early stages following the TBI these individuals may be identified with language of confusion or typical aphasia. There is some evidence indicating that individuals with right hemisphere damage from a CHI tend to be more like language of confusion than left hemisphere-damaged individuals with CHI. The TBI may also result in concurrent speech (dysarthria) and swallowing (dysphagia) disorders as well.

Sometimes it is easier to characterize the cognitive and communication symptoms according to the four phases in recovery from the TBI:

1. *Coma phase* where there is loss of consciousness lasting from hours to weeks; this period is also considered as "vegetative state." The obvious clinical manifestation is the inability to arouse or obtain a response to any form of stimulation. The duration of coma is used to determine prognosis for recovery however, no specific demarcation points are established in the available literature.

2. *Posttraumatic amnesia (PTA) phase* begins with gain of consciousness and ends with the ability to remember daily events with signs of progressive improvement in orientation. This stage is marked by obvious impairment in the language modalities with ample examples of linguistic symptoms that permit assignment of such individuals to one of the typical aphasia classification categories;

frequently, the assignment to language of confusion is appropriate for individuals at this stage of recovery.

3. *Rapid recovery phase,* when significant progress occurs over a few months (3–6) depending on severity of the injury; there is a dramatic improvement in language-specific symptoms.

4. *Long-term plateau phase,* the final stage when there is the persistence of residual communication deficits highlighted by pragmatic problems and higher level cognitive symptoms. The recovery of prevailing symptoms appears to slow down or even show signs of plateau.

Right Hemisphere Injury (RHI)

The prominent clinical feature is damage to the right hemisphere, which is considered nondominant for language functions based on sodium amytol injections (or Wada technique) in 85 percent of individuals. This fact indicates that majority of individuals with RHI show no obvious signs of aphasia yet they encounter subtle linguistic and cognitive problems, which has resulted in segregating this group of individuals under a unique cognitive-communication disorder.

Perceptual symptoms representing agnosia highlight this category. Some of the possible agnosias associated with RHI include anosognosia, prosopagnosia, agraphagnosia (inability to recognize letters and numbers), visual-spatial problems and amusia. The prevailing visual agnosias may be compounded by the presence of hemianopia and constructional apraxia as well. The linguistic problems in RHI may be seen for the parameters of pragmatics, semantic and phonology. Pragmatically, their verbal output may be characterized by irrelevancy and topic-focus disorganization, and these symptoms may be evident during sequential narration and via response impulsivity. Word retrieval problems account for the semantic breakdown, and the presence of verbal apraxia albeit mild in severity, explain the phonological errors. Sometimes the phonological problems are embedded within the overt dysarthric and dysprosodic speech productions.

Individuals with RHI also show evidence of higher order cognitive-communication problems through impaired comprehension and ex-ecutive functions particularly with emotional content. Some examples include difficulty interpreting (understanding) the prosodic features of a verbal message, as well as recognizing emotions, humor and metaphoric aspects of language. Individuals with RHI tend to show no difficulty recognizing different emotions (angry, sad, happy, and surprise) in isolation, but they have greater difficulty clustering sets of negative emotions. When making judgments regarding emotionality of the presented stimuli, these individuals depend on the variable of *duration* (timing) to make auditory judgments while those with left hemisphere damage attend to the feature of fundamental frequency (Fo) variability (pitch inflection) in their interpretation of the same stimuli (Van Lancker & Sidtis, 1992).

It needs to be noted that acquisition of aphasia is also possible following a RHI among left-handed individuals, and similarly crossed aphasia should not be ruled out as well. In such instances the individual with RHI is more likely to be assigned to one of the established apahsia classification categories.

Language of Confusion aka Organic Brain Dysfunction

Approximately six percent of acutely brain-damaged patients fall in this category. Some common identifiers from their medical history include a sudden onset of brain damage from one of the possible etiologies: head trauma, nonocclusive ischemic CVA, anoxia, tumor, TIA, metabolic disturbance, drug dependency, or immediately following a coronary surgery. The site of lesion tends to be nonspecific regarding the involvement of either the right or the left hemisphere; however, there is some evidence of prefrontal (ventromedial) lesion and its linkage with the limbic system. Typically, language of confusion is associated with younger or middle age groups.

Their performance on language tests may fall in the normal or near normal range particularly for the structured (convergent) tasks. Linguistically, their verbal output is fluent with primarily pragmatic problems that are characterized by irrelevancy (noncoherency), tangential responses, confabulations, verbosity, and semantically empty speech (Drummond, 1986). Although their verbal fluency and corresponding linguistic error patterns may resemble characteristics of Wernicke's aphasia, individuals with language of confusion distinguish themselves by showing little or no evidence of comprehension problem. These individuals demonstrate breakdown in perceptual and cognitive functions that are observed as attention, orientation, perception, STM and executive function (abstraction) problems. Their perceptual problems are highlighted by the presence of visual agnosia and visuospatial disorientation. Examples of abstraction problems are observed during activities requiring sequencing events, problem solving, performing calculations, explaining connotation/metaphors, and judging emotions. Sometimes these individuals have been described as emotionally flat and show signs of visual hallucinations as well.

Individuals with language of confusion differ from other fluent aphasias such as Wernicke's aphasia based on their relative differences in site of lesion and relatively intact auditory comprehension. The obvious pragmatic and executive function problems of this group also differentiate them from the fluent anomic aphasia. Their ability to successfully complete structured tasks without progressive decline in quality distinguishes them from individuals with dementia. The best news is their fair-to-good prognosis for recovery.

Dementia/Language of Generalized Intellectual Impairment/Organic Brain Syndrome

Dementia is an acquired condition that encompasses myriad etiologies and disease. It is an umbrella term that is reflective of decline in cognitive functions of auditory and/or visual perception, memory, executive functions of reasoning and abstraction, as well as the language modalities of comprehension and production. Each of these characteristics defines dementia as a cognitive-communication disorder. The multiplicity and severity of the impaired cognitive and linguistic skills depend on the underlying neurological disease which tend to be neurodegenerative in nature (see Table 5.1, p. 77).

Several types of classifications are used to reflect the medical data surrounding the dementia. One dichotomy relates to the nature of the neuropathology: reversible or irreversible. *Reversible dementia* implies that the observed symptoms may be alleviated or reversed to normalcy, while *irreversible dementia* indicates that the disorder will continue to progress in severity and diversity over time irrespective of intervention. The second categorization focuses on the site of origin of the neurological disease that is responsible for the observed dementia and it clusters them according to *cortical, subcortical,* and *mixed (combined cortical* and *subcortical) dementia.* If the degeneration is cortical in origin, then the initial communication breakdown may be reflective of either aphasia or dementia. In subcortical degeneration, the symptoms of dementia may occur only in the late/advanced stages of the diseased condition; some examples of such degenerative diseases include Parkinson's disease, Huntington's disease, and progressive supranuclear palsy. Another categorization, *vascular versus nonvascular dementia,* directs attention to reduced cerebral blood flow as the trigger factor; vascular dementia is most often associated with multiple CVAs (or "multi-infarct" dementia). Sometimes *senile versus presenile dementia* is used to distinguish the age of onset of the dementia. Typically, presenile dementia is determined if the cognitive-communication disorder is recognized in individuals under 65 years; this category is occasionally referred under frontal lobe dementia. The only term, *progressive aphasia* (or *primary progressive aphasia*), focuses on breakdown in communication; it has been used to characterize patients with progressive neurological diseases who show selective, and primary, decline in language functions during the early stages of neurodegeneration.

Clinically, the most relevant approach to dementia classification is the determination of the clustering of the communication and cognitive symptoms. The most popular neuropsychological format, the Global Deterioration Scale, assigns the individual to one of seven stages of dementia (Reisberg, Ferris, DeLeon & Crook, 1982). Progressive degradation of language or communication functions however, is described through three stages (early, middle and late). A summary of the defining characteristics according to each of these severity-based classifications is provided in Table 8.2. It needs to be noted that language-related, or aphasic-like symptoms are prevalent whenever dementia results from cortical lesions. In contrast, speech-related (dysarthric) symptoms predominate in subcortical lesions. Concurrent motor problems such as gait disturbances and sensory problems associated with the aging process (visual problems/presbyopia and hearing disorders/presbycusis) can exacerbate the symptoms of dementia.

Finally, two important clues can be gleaned when assessing individuals with dementia. First, they show relatively better performance on tasks that are presented earlier in the session. Second, these individuals demonstrate steep degradation in performance for lengthy or complex tasks and stimuli within, and between, the different subtest areas.

Table 8.2. Linguistic and Cognitive Symptoms Characterizing the Different Stages of Dementia (adapted from Reisberg, et al, 1982).

Stages of Dementia	Linguistic Symptoms	Cognitive Symptoms
I: No cognitive decline	No obvious problem	No obvious problem
II: Very mild cognitive decline	Subjective reports of anomia	Subjective reports of memory problems/ forgetfulness
III: Mild cognitive decline	Comprehension & pragmatic functions preserved Successful communication in casual & routine conversation Increased verbosity & verbal irrelevancies Mildly impaired performance on language tests Fluent verbal output with word-finding problems Resembles Anomic aphasia	Some STM problem Some concentration problem Denial of symptoms
IV: Moderate cognitive decline (late confusional phase)	Mild comprehension problems Obvious pragmatic problems during conversation (impaired turn taking, incoherent, confabulatory) Fluent verbal output Mild syntactical & phonological problems (semantic jargon/empty speech evident) Resemble Wernicke's aphasia	Increased concentration & STM problems Difficulty with complex reasoning tasks Withdrawal from challenging situations Increased denial of symptoms Flattening affect/emotional dullness

Table 8.2 – *Continued*

Stages of Dementia	Linguistic Symptoms	Cognitive Symptoms
V: Moderately severe cognitive decline (phase of early dementia)	Decreased participation in communication Nonfluent verbal output (limited & telegrammatic) Need constant cues Presence of phonemic paraphasia & dysarthria	Disorientation to time, person & place Acalculia present Needs assistance for routine activities Impaired judgment skills LTM problems emerge
VI. Severe cognitive decline (middle phase dementia)	Decline in comprehension performance Severe impairment for all 4 linguistic parameters Little or no verbal output Verbal stereotypes & echolalia may be present Resembles global aphasia	Increased agitation to least provocation Increased attention problems Marked LTM problems
VII: Very severe cognitive decline (late dementia)	Noncommunicative (mutism) Vegetative (involuntary) vocalization present	Requires total assistance

APHASIA VERSUS
COGNITIVE-COMMUNICATION DISORDERS

There are obvious similarities in symptom manifestations as a consequence of brain damage irrespective of the diverse etiologies or the nature of the lesion. Similarities among individuals with brain damage help appreciate the fact that different language symptoms are interrelated because of their interdependent neural connections. The commonality of some symptoms among these different groups of disorders makes it feasible to share the diagnostic tools for assessing them, and to also apply some common intervention strategies for their management irrespective of the etiology of the brain damage.

The paradox of commonalities among the clinical categories is the plausibility of heightened confusion among the different types of linguistic-communication disorders. This section therefore highlights some of the influencing factors that help to differentiate the syndrome of aphasia from cognitive-communication disorders:

- Etiology: Generally individuals with first episode ischemic (occlusive) CVA are classified as one of the aphasias, while those with TBI or a degenerative neurological disease (progressive lesions) may be assigned to cognitive-communication disorders. Individuals with right hemisphere lesions may show characteristics of either aphasia or a cognitive-communication disorder.

- Site and location of lesion: This factor can be dichotomized in several ways. It can be referred as specific (or focal) or nonspecific (or general/diffuse) lesion, or as single versus multiple lesions, right versus left (language-dominant) hemispheric lesion, or as a cortical versus subcortical lesion. Of these possibilities, individuals with left hemisphere damage are classified under the aphasia while those with right (nondominant) hemisphere lesions are generally highlighted as a unique group of cognitive-communication disorder.

- Time since onset (or duration) of the brain damage is another consideration. Acutely ill patients, immediately after incurring the brain damage, sometimes conform less readily to established aphasia classifications because the effect of diaschisis may invoke symptoms and behaviors that defy such categorization. This possibility has resulted in the frequent designation to the language of confusion category for acute patients.

- Chronological age: Typically older individuals with ischemic CVA are readily classified to the aphasic categories than younger adults with similar etiologies; this is perhaps due to the differences in the overall integrity of their respective physiological systems. Furthermore, younger individuals often acquire brain damage from other etiologies, which accounts for their frequent assignment to cognitive-communication disorders.
- Previous/concurrent medical history: Co-existing conditions such as diabetes, hypertension, coronary disease, depression and having undergone a recent surgery tend to exacerbate the presence and severity of the observed symptoms. This reality is further clouded by the fact that these individuals may take a regimen of medications, between 6–10 different prescriptions. The net effect of their vulnerable physiological systems imposes a clinical challenge for determining a precise classificatory assignment, and at times it is expedient to consider such individuals under one of the cognitive-communication disorders.
- Concurrent perceptual problems: Prevailing and obvious perceptual impairments can compound the diagnostic process. Generally, individuals demonstrating a preponderance of perceptual problems tend to be assigned to one of the cognitive-communication disorders. For example, one or more types of agnosias are prevalent in right hemisphere lesions, while persistent and progressive disorientation present as the primary symptoms of language of confusion or dementia.
- Linguistic symptoms: Obvious disruption in pragmatic skills is typically associated with cognitive-communication disorders than for aphasia. This is perhaps because pragmatic functions describe the adequacy of interactive/social communication which is the primary concern for individuals with cognitive-communication disorders. In contrast, aphasic verbal output reflects disbursement of error patterns across all four linguistic parameters; this explains the detailed scrutiny of the nature of breakdown in each of the four linguistic parameters for aphasia as discussed in Chapters 6 and 7. Regarding verbal fluency, individuals with cognitive-communication problems, particularly those with TBI, RHI, and language of confusion, tend to be fluent; those with aphasia and dementia may show different degrees of verbal fluency.
- Clinician competency: Clinical expertise in acquired neurogenic

communication disorders is an evolutionary process and errors are possible in a novice. It is well established that complex tasks are difficult for all patients and that the linguistic parameter of semantics (reflecting word retrieval) is impaired in all individuals with cerebral lesions. An astute clinician considers this factor in the selection of an assessment protocol, and with careful scrutiny of obtained performances determines possible interrelationships between responses, parses global from esoteric symptoms; this vigilance is vital in accurate interpretation of test results and in preventing possible misdiagnosis of the communication disorder. Table 8.3 is a composite of the different factors that contribute to successful differential diagnosis for linguistic and cognitive-communication disorders; this chart is provided as a guidance to sensitize the clinician regarding the interplay among these factors.

PROGNOSTIC VARIABLES

The term *prognosis* refers to the speculation regarding the course of recovery or outcome of a problem, which in this instance relates to communication. It is important to bear in mind that one of the most important feature of the majority of acquired communication disorders is that they are "temporary" in nature. The determination of prognosis for a neurogenic communication disorder is important because it influences the decision regarding recommending an individual for treatment/rehabilitation; thus, prognosis is discussed in the context of "rehabilitation potential." Several endogenous and exogenous factors contribute toward estimation of prognosis for language/communication recovery. Some examples of endogenous prognostic factors include the following:

- *Etiology:* The nature of brain damage directly influences the degree of recovery. Individuals with nonprogressive diseases such as TBI or CVA have better prognosis than those with progressive cerebral lesions from degenerative neurological diseases or advanced brain tumor. The nonprogressive forms of brain damage also tend to be sudden in onset while symptoms resulting from brain tumors and degenerative diseases such as Alzheimer's disease tend to be gradual in onset. Among the nonprogressive lesions, individuals with ischemic CVA tend to stabilize sooner

Table 8.3. Differential Diagnosis between Aphasia and Four Cognitive Communication Disorders.

	Aphasia	Language of Confusion	TBI	RHI	Dementia
Medical information					
Onset	Sudden	Sudden	Sudden	Sudden	Gradual
Etiology	Any	Any	Trauma	Any	Any
Lesion site	Variable	Variable	Variable	Variable	Variable
Age	Any	Young/middle	Young/middle	Any	Middle/old
Language information					
Test performance (degree of difficulty)	Variable	Normal/mild	Progressive-poor	Normal/mild	Variable
Verbal output	Fluent/nonfluent	Fluent	Fluent/nonfluent	Fluent	Fluent→nonfluent
Pragmatic problem	Yes/no	Yes	Yes/no	Yes/no	Yes: progressive
Word retrieval	Yes	Yes	Yes	Yes/no	Yes: progressive
Cognitive information					
Attention problem	Yes/No	Yes	Yes/no	No	Yes
Perceptual problem	No/mild	Yes/no	Yes/no	Yes	Yes?
STM problem	Yes?	Yes	Yes?	No	Yes
Abstraction problem	Yes?	Yes	Yes	Yes	Yes
Behavioral information					
Emotional affect	Normal	Abnormal	Normal/abnormal	Abnormal	Abnormal
Prognosis	Variable	Fair/good	Fair/good	Fair/good	Poor

than those with head trauma in terms of their recovery curves; the individuals with TBI may continue to show improvement across a longer period. Generally, there is no clinical difference in recovery trends between OHI and CHI if there is damage to the primary language areas in the dominant hemisphere. Of the different ischemic CVAs those with hemorrhagic CVA tend to show relatively less recovery, or plateau within six months postonset, while individuals with embolic CVA may continue to recover beyond this period.

- *Chronological age:* The brain's capacity to reorganize, or *cerebral plasticity,* is optimal from infancy to early adolescence; thereafter, it is capable of some degree of *adaptive plasticity* throughout life. It is a fact that younger individuals show greater amount of recovery in relatively shorter time period and therefore, they tend to have better prognosis. Demographics also show that there is a likelihood of a greater number and magnitude of symptoms with advancing age. It is commonly considered that individuals under 60 years have better prognosis. The variable of age however, also interacts with etiology since the majority of younger adults acquire the brain damage from TBI.

- *Lesion data:* Individuals with initial/single episode of brain damage have better prognosis than those with multiple lesions. Lesions involving the left (language dominant) hemisphere have poorer prognosis for recovery than those with nondominant, right hemisphere lesions. An equally important factor is size of lesion; individuals with larger lesions tend to show less recovery than those with smaller infarctions. Location of lesion also plays a role in language recovery. Cortical lesions involving the gray matter of the language processing zone show less recovery than medial white matter lesions near the same language areas; also, language-related symptoms resulting from subcortical lesions show better resolution than those occurring as a consequence of cortical lesions. Finally, a well-circumscribed, focal lesion has relatively better prognosis than a diffused or generalized lesion.

- *Medical history:* Premorbid or concurrent medical conditions may affect recovery and limit or contraindicate specific forms of intervention. Some examples of medical conditions that may impede recovery include coronary and pulmonary disease, hypertension, diabetes, cancer, musculoskeletal diseases (arthritis and orthopedic problems), severe psychiatric diseases, and other neurological diseases. A previous history of brain damage from either TBI or ischemic CVA can increase the person's vulnerability for subsequent brain damage and exacerbate the prevailing symptoms. Also, previous history of brain damage from either TBI or ischemic CVA can increase a person's vulnerability for subsequent brain damage and this exacerbate the prevailing symptoms.

- *Duration since brain damage:* Also referred as time postonset, this prognostic factor favors individuals with recent onset or acute patients than those who are chronic. This distinction however, should not be confused with determination of in- or outpatient status. Although acute patients may appear more severe due to the effect of *diaschisis* because the damaged area deprives the surrounding healthy areas from performing their routine functions, these individuals tend to show significant recovery as the suppressed remote areas gradually regain their functions in the early months following the brain damage. This improvement is termed as *spontaneous recovery,* which is defined as the period of physiological restitution immediately following the onset of brain damage during which there is dramatic recovery of various neurological and speech-language functions. Spontaneous recovery is also referred as the second stage recovery and typically, it is considered to occur between 0–6 months after the damage; this period may be extended in some persons because different individuals recover at different physiological rates thus displaying their unique pattern of spontaneous recovery. Some of the physiological events reflecting the internal adjustments and stabilization that explain spontaneous recovery include the following factors:
  1. Tissue disintegration or removal of infarcted neural tissue.
  2. Reduction of local and/or generalized edema to help the healthy tissue resume its suppressed metabolic activity.
  3. Vascular adjustment through resorption of the hematoma or small hemorrhage can occur; this is usually more effective in fresh blood clots. Also possible is *lysis of emboli,* which is the disintegration of the occlusive agent within the artery. This event results in *recanalization,* or reopening of the lumen of the blood vessel. Both lysis and recanalization generally show up as local recovery. Evidence from angiograms performed immediately after the onset of brain damage and then one year later, sup-

ports the occurrence of recanalization and reduction in the number of occluded branches in the majority of patients. Another vascular change is the establishment of *collateral circulation,* which is the formation of new vessels (or collaterals) from adjacent healthy arteries at the edge of the infarcted area to help direct oxygen to the affected region. This phenomenon is also reported as the *effect of normal interarterial anastomosis.*

4. Neural reorganization through *nerve sprouting* is a sort of restructuring or rewiring between neurons to reactivate disrupted synaptic connections. This concept is illustrated in Figure 8.2 where a healthy adjacent neuron ('C') may send collateral to reactivate the "widowed" neuron ('B') that has been deprived of neural signals because of its connection with the damaged area ('A'). The formation of nerve sprouting is facilitated by NGF in the astrocytes. Another example of neural reorganization is seen through the activation of latent (or underused) silent synapses to assume the functions of the damaged ones. Each of these neural changes reflects compensation of the impaired functions by undamaged areas; the basis for this indication is further supported by the fact that synapses are constantly rearranged in normal nonbrain-damaged individuals as well. Overt signs of neural reorganization are reflected when there is a change in muscle tone or a behavioral response following brain damage.

5. Neurogenesis or birth of new neurons is also possible. Recent reports indicate that "stem-like" or immature (undifferentiated) cells have been found in the adult cerebellum and near the olfactory bulb. These stem cells tend to be amorphous and flat, lacking the axons and dendrite of mature neurons. Under normal conditions these cells would rapidly differentiate into specialized cells, assume neuronal functions and would no longer reproduce themselves. However, treating them with a protein called epidermal growth factor (EGF) has shown to develop these cells into neurons, astrocytes, and oligodendrocytes. Once neuronal differentiation results, these cells no longer act like stem cells and they spread into the surrounding regions. Their tendency to migrate to the damaged areas as neurons and oligodendrocytes is verified in laboratory animal models (mice).

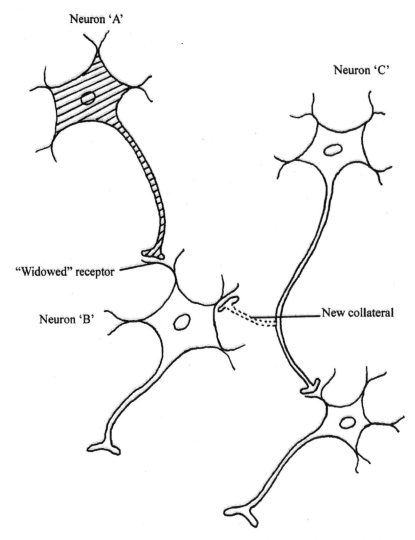

Figure 8.2. Physiological recovery resulting from neural reorganization: dead neuron 'A', widowed neuron 'B', and donor neuron 'C'.

- Type and severity of aphasia is also considered as a prognostic variable. As expected, individuals with the least number of symptoms, or anomic aphasia, have optimal prognosis and recovery. Similarly, those with crossed aphasia tend to have relatively better prognosis because of their utilization of multiple, alternative circuitries for language functions. Also, individuals who have relatively intact auditory comprehension ability tend to have better prognosis; thus Broca's aphasia has better prognosis than Wernicke's aphasia, while those with global aphasia have the worst prognosis. Finally, Wernicke's aphasia without (neologistic) jargon has better prognosis than that with jargon.

- Concurrent sensory and perceptual impairments may exacerbate the communication problem and therefore, adversely influence prognosis. For example, a peripheral hearing or vision loss may affect performance for auditory or visual comprehension, respectively. Similarly, hemianopia and agnosia may also complicate the comprehension abilities among these individuals.
- Motor deficits such as the presence of hemiplegia have no obvious relationship to recovery of language or communication functions. Such problems may however, affect the legibility of handwriting skills and interfere when writing is required for self-expression.
- Associated behavioral symptoms, described in Chapter 6, may retard progress and recovery. Interference from an isolated symptom may be distracting but manageable during intervention; however, occurrence of multiple symptoms as a cluster may create obstacles for achieving successful communication outcome.
- Preferred laterality/handedness: Individuals who show a preference for left-handedness have better prognosis because of the possibility that they may utilize both hemispheres for language functions. These individuals frequently represent crossed aphasia as well.
- Gender: Traditional literature clearly favors females regarding prognosis because their vascular system is healthier than the male cohorts. Contemporary life and working styles however, has narrowed this divide so that females are just as vulnerable as males to any of the etiologies and associated consequences of brain damage.
- Lifestyle preferences, personality and motivation: Persistence of personal habits such as smoking, alcohol consumption, or use of recreational drugs/substance abuse even after the brain damage is detriment to recovery and thus contributes to unfavorable prognosis. Similarly, low level of motivation for self-improvement may adversely affect recovery and rehabilitation outcome; perseverance and positive attitude toward overcoming physiological and physical setbacks is definitely an endogenous asset. Poor

motivation level may be inferred through noncompliancy when implementing therapeutic strategies, unexcused absences from therapy, lack of nonmaintenance of a prescribed schedule for daily activities, and refusal to participate in routine or structured tasks/activities.

There are some exogenous variables that can also influence prognosis and recovery, and they include the following:

- Educational history does not show a clear bias toward prognosis for recovery, however the variable of literacy is relevant since it influences reading and writing performances. The integrity of these two modalities may enhance recovery since they have the potential to serve as adjuncts to enhance the impaired listening and speaking modalities.

- Occupation: An individual's profession or occupation is not an obvious determiner for prognosis. This factor is significant if the victim has sufficient assurance of resuming the pre-morbid employment even after the brain damage; this prospective may provide extra incentive and reinforcement to strive for recovery.

- Nature of therapy: There is clear evidence that initiation of therapy immediately after the onset of brain damage has very favorable outcome. Another important factor is the type and intensity of the therapy. Evidence-based research indicates that a comprehensive treatment plan that focuses on minimizing the impaired symptoms through both facilitative and compensatory strategies has beneficial effects even in the presence of severe communication impairments. In contrast, utilization of prescriptive programmed intervention does not show improvement in impaired behaviors and functions.

- Contextual factors include several environmental conditions that can influence recovery. One of them relates to level of personal independence pertaining to domicile. An individual who resides independently has a greater incentive to recover and maintain personal autonomy than one in a community living environment (long-term facility). Similarly, family or social support can contribute to favorable prognosis. The individual with attentive caregivers who provide stimulation, encouragement and time tend to show greater recovery and better outcome.

SUMMARY

The prominent features of a communication disorder are displayed in similar fashion in one's native language irrespective of cultural differences and methods of communication. In this respect the concept of linguistic universals is attested among individuals with brain damage as well. These individuals also display distinct clusters of symptoms that segregate them into obscure categories such as aphasia and cognitive-communication disorders. The linkage between symptoms poses a clinical challenge for making accurate diagnosis of the type and severity of the communication disorder; this calls for critical integration of underlying knowledge of interacting psycho- and neurolinguistic factors with observed clinical performances. A dynamic clinician is also required to maintain active vigilance to rule out related disorders and derive at a precise diagnosis–the outcome of this exercise is successful differential diagnosis.

Chapter 9

LINGUISTIC-COMMUNICATION INTERVENTION

The primary definition of *rehabilitation* is "to return to normal," and a less exacting interpretation is "to return to useful service." These descriptions can mean as much as running a company or just planning tomorrow's wardrobe; each of these concerns are of equal importance to respective victims of brain damage. Rehabilitation programs for adults with language/communication disorders began toward the end of World War II due an influx of veterans with traumatic brain injuries. Since the late 1940s treatment approaches implemented through individualized sessions or in group therapy have embraced several schools of thought. Irrespective of the approach, there is a call for constant interplay between two parallel treatment objectives, *facilitation* or improvement in impaired symptoms and *compensation* or circumventing the prevailing symptoms.

This chapter is devoted to noninvasive, behavioral treatment approaches for adults with acquired aphasia and cognitive-communication disorders. It provides salient information on different components that are essential for an effective communication-related intervention. The content also directs attention to pertinent treatment variables, and distinguishes between treatment versus management, and between individual versus group intervention. Finally, it discusses efficacy issues not only to justify intervention but also highlight an optimistic outcome for the majority of individuals with linguistic and cognitive-communication disorders.

Table 9.1. Applicable Treatment Approaches for the Different Categories of Neurogenic Communication Disorders.

Treatment approach	Aphasia	Language of confusion	Traumatic brain injury	Right hemisphere injury	Dementia
Didactic	Yes	–	Yes	–	–
Behavior modification	Yes	Yes	Yes	Yes	–
Stimulation	Yes	Yes	Yes	Yes	Yes
Association	Yes	Yes	Yes	Yes	Yes
Functional reorganization	Yes	Yes	Yes	Yes	Yes?
Neurolinguistic	Yes	Yes	Yes	–	–
Pragmatic	Yes	Yes	Yes	Yes	Yes
Cognitive neuropsychological	–	–	Yes	–	–

TREATMENT APPROACHES

Behavioral intervention is founded on the fact that the brain is *plastic,* indicating that it is able to change and adapt itself based on enriching sensory and motor activities. The majority of contributions to management of linguistic-communication disorders have evolved from treatment of individuals with aphasia and TBI (Howard & Hatfield, 1987), however, they are applicable to other disorders as well (see Table 9.1). It is important to remember that treatment approaches and philosophies help understand and appreciate the rationale underlying different aspects of intervention. Therefore, this section is a summary of each of the major schools of thought relating to intervention of neurogenic communication disorders.

Didactic Approach

The oldest approach, since the nineteenth century, relies on common sense and intuition, and it is based on the premise that language is "retaught." It applies traditional patterns of teaching reading, writing and grammar that are commonly used with school children and nonnative English speakers, to treat adults with communication disorders as well. This approach directs the clinician to assume the primary responsibility for selecting a prescriptive curriculum (content) from available resources, and ensures its effective delivery. In the United States, Jon Eisenson applied the principles of didactic therapy through group intervention with veterans of World War II.

Behavior Modification (or Operant) Approach

This approach contends that language is "relearned" and it is derived from the principles from behavioral psychology including Pavlov's operant conditioning and Skinner's stimulus-response models. It focuses on "how" select skills or behaviors are learned, and advocates systematic steps toward modifying or minimizing unacceptable (impaired) behaviors. Simultaneously, it pays close attention to delivering appropriate reinforcement of acceptable (target) behaviors. Behavior modification ideology guarantees a gradual decline in impairment with a corresponding incline in improvement (recovery). This approach is widely used in clinical practice, and its applications are numerous: any form of individualized step-by-step intervention program utilizes the principles of behavior modification.

Stimulation Approach

The term "stimulation" implies careful manipulation of input (sensory) modalities and provision of intensified delivery of stimuli through the selected channels(s). This approach aims to regain access to language functions via enhanced presentation of a stimulus through either a single (*unimodal*) or several (*multimodal*) sensory systems. Both unimodal and multimodal forms of stimulation may be delivered in a systematized protocol (or *specific stimulation*), or they may be implemented in a nonstructured format or situation (or *nonspecific stimulation*); the common understanding is that the patient/client does not have to be an active (obligatory) participant during any form of stimulation. A popular application of specific stimulation is the coma stimulation protocols delivered to unresponsive individuals who receive a series of uni- or multimodal stimulation to evoke an acceptable, or even irrelevant, overt response. Nonspecific stimulation is frequently referred as environmental stimulation or socialization therapy where the individual is exposed to all or any possible stimulation from radio or television broadcasts, or persons in the immediate environment.

A prominent advocate of *language stimulation,* or *auditory stimulation* approach, was Hildred Schuell (1964) who emphasized use of exogenous, multimodal stimulation to arouse and reorganize the impaired language processes. Schuell contended that parallel stimulation of all (both impaired and intact) modalities result in a summation effect because this format serves to reinforce each of the participating sensory systems; she also considered multimodal stimulation as a pre-requisite toward restoring the impaired output modalities. Schuell's multimodal stimulation primarily includes the auditory system in conjunction with visual and/or tactile senses perhaps for the following reasons:
- The auditory (listening) modality plays a major role in routine verbal communication because it helps comprehend the delivered message to perpetuate the interaction.
- All verbal speakers learn their first (or native) language via the auditory system therefore it is natural for a patient to favor this sensory modality despite its disruption.
- Clinically, assessment results show that there is some preservation of at least one sensory modality even in the most severely brain

damaged individual; this reality justifies use of the residual system to gain access to the dysfunctional brain.

Schuell suggests that intervention should involve all levels within the auditory modality through systematic progression from lower to higher order cognitive functions:

Attention (listening)

↓

Recognition (localization)

↓

Perception (discrimination)

↓

Comprehension (understanding)

(

Association (integration with other systems)

↓

LTM (storage and retention)

One application of multimodal, specific stimulation is reflected in Rosenbek's (1985) "Integral Stimulation" method for apraxia of speech, which describes systematic clinician-delivered steps during multimodal ("watch and listen") presentation.

Contemporary evidence regarding the brain's increased reliance on vision has given precedence for including visual stimulation in therapy as well. Furthermore, the indication of reciprocity between visual and tactile sensations known as *sensory-cross connection,* replaces the traditional static view of the brain and provides physiological endorsement for multimodal stimulation.

Association Approach

Joseph Wepman (1951) incorporated the principles of stimulation to focus on language facilitation and association. He contended that an effective intervention should (1) result in lowered threshold for the response or induce *facilitation,* and (2) it should be prepared to modify any stimulus to create the opportunity for making some *association* (a compensatory strategy) with the target. Wepman applied the stimulation and response elicitation phases through the concept of "shutter" principle, which equates the brain to a camera lens. Accordingly, he described the brain/shutter to operate in three hierarchical stages:

1. The shutter opens whenever the patient receives the stimulus.

Successful delivery of this stage depends on stimulus appropriateness (familiarity, frequency of use, complexity), its perceptual adequacy, and clinician presentation style (rate, clarity). I think a parallel can be made between Wepman's three stages and the neurophysiology of cellular excitation; this first stage event appears to be analogous to the subliminal stage of depolarization.

2. The shutter closes while the patient is absorbing the stimulus. In addition to the stimulus characteristics required for Stage 1, this stage also relies on adequate imposition of response (processing) time. This event may be considered analogous to the graded potential (subliminal continual stimulation) phase of neuronal stimulation.

3. The shutter reopens when the patient is ready to respond, or if the patient asks for further input (assistance). Successful response, or outcome of this stage, depends on factors such as the strength of the stimulus, its effective presentation and instructions, as well as the interstimulus latency (or pacing the presentation). Neurophysiologically, this stage can be equated to the generation of an action potential.

Unfortunately, Wepman retracted his emphasis on direct, language-oriented intervention during his later years (1972). His shutter principle however, makes sense in the context of later studies on cortical evoked potentials. The three hierarchical steps utilize the principles of operant conditioning and are indeed valid for effective treatment delivery; one may caution however, that improper handling of Stages 2 and 3 may precipitate unacceptable behaviors like perseveration, frustration, or even a catastrophic reaction. Such inappropriate occurrences are possible if the stimuli are presented at too fast a pace or there is insufficient time between successive stimulations. Neurophysiologically, perseveration may be a manifestation of the need for longer refractory period because the damaged system does not appear to keep up with the pace of stimulus presentation. According to Luria (1980) however, perseveration is a reflection of "pathological inertia" meaning that there is persistent after effects of excitation (stimulation) for an abnormally long period.

The principle of "association" is frequently applied in treatment delivery. A common example is use of cues to foster connections with a target response/behavior; cues can be self-initiated (revision or repetition of a response) or they can be exogenous if they are delivered by a clinician or caregiver. Multimodal stimulations result in sensory integration which also symbolizes the concept of association between the activated sensory modalities. Another example of association theory is a grammatically complete sentence, which is rich in linguistic attributes that provide paradigmatic (relationship between syllables or between phonological and syntactical units) and syntagmatic (relationships between semantic units) associations (Jakobson & Halle, 1956).

Functional (Neurological) Reorganization Approach

This approach has been popular in Eastern Europe and Russia since the World War II. Proponents affirm that although the brain damage is irreversible, it is possible to reorganize the disrupted functions. The focus of this approach is to uncover and activate relatively intact, and perhaps unpopular or inaccessible, cortical areas and use them for communication. Alexander Romanovich Luria (1980) who was a primary advocate of this approach contended that reorganization (or recovery) of damaged functions is possible because of two physiological mechanisms:

- homologous regions of the contralateral (nondamaged) hemisphere assume the functions that are impaired due to the damaged areas; and
- functional systems are *plastic* (moldable) to allow new, or uncommitted, areas to learn the impaired functions and incorporate them with their own functions.

Luria advocates two forms of strategies for successful functional reorganization:

1. *Intrasystemic reorganization,* which is an attempt to improve a function (or response) within the target modality by manipulating the same system. This principle is applied whenever the clinician shifts the focus from an incorrect response to seek a lower, or another level within the same modality that can yield a correct response. For example, the client may be directed to repeat the target word if unable to provide its name; in this instance the response was altered from naming to repetition, but the expectation of eliciting a verbal response was maintained. This form of reorganization is also utilized when providing cues that share some characteristics with the target response or modality (e.g.,

semantic or phonological cue to help retrieve the target word). The clinician can also develop a cue hierarchy by first presenting a relatively less informative, or semantic cue (e.g., "animal" or "barks" if the target is "dog") and then proceed to offering a specific phonemic/initial syllable cue (e.g., "da" for "dog"). Some examples of practical applications of intrasystemic reorganization are provided in Table 9.2.

2. *Intersystemic reorganization* utilizes a less impaired system either in conjunction with, or in place of, the impaired modality. Some examples include encouraging the use of a hand gesture or provide the response in written form to compensate for a verbal output problem; or combine an auditory instruction with a related visual stimulus or cue in the form of a picture, written word or gesture when encountering a breakdown in auditory comprehension (see Table 9.2).

The concept of *deblocking* is sometimes used in place of these two forms of compensatory reorganization. It is defined as the use of less impaired system(s) to eliminate a "blockage" created by the impaired system, and thus circumvent (or bypass) the impaired system. This concept is incorporated in esoteric treatment methods such as the "Melodic Intonation Therapy," "Drawing for Communication" and "Visual Action Therapy" (Helm-Estabrooks & Albert, 2004), as well as the *Amerind* hand gestures (Skelly, 1979).

It is important to review the assessment data and verify two factors prior to selecting either intra- or intersystemic reorganization strategies. One of these includes the firm understanding of the least and most impaired systems; this information is crucial when considering intersystemic strategies. The second factor pertains to determining the levels or tasks that are relatively easy, and difficult, within each modality; this is vital for selecting intrasystemic strategies during intervention. Clinicians offer each of these options as exogenous strategies when the objective is to modify an inaccurate response, or if the goal is to further refine the client's performance. The client may also employ them as endogenous strategies when attempting to communicate; some examples include revising a word or repeating a word (intrasystemic) when confronting a word finding problem, or using hand gestures (intersystemic) when communicating a message (see Table 9.2).

Table 9.2. Examples of Intrasystemic and Intersystemic Reorganization Strategies for the Two Primary Language Modalities.

Modality	Intrasystemic	Intersystemic
Auditory Comprehension	Present information at a slower rate Increase stress placement on key words Combine gestures with verbal instructions	Show important picture or written word Provide the instructions in written form
Verbal Expression	Repeat or revise the target word Provide a semantic cue Provide a phonemic/initial syllable cue Repeat the same word several times Speak in a singing tone Recite numbers and words in a sequential order Proved one-word response for entire sentence Encourage use of circumlocutions	Write the target word (instead of speaking) Point to the target picture or word Read the target word Tap toes or clap when speaking Draw the target object or action Use gestures

Neurolinguistic Approach

This approach incorporates neurological information regarding site of lesion with observed linguistic symptoms such as agrammatism, paragrammatism, anomia, etc. It establishes treatment objectives based on three considerations: (1) linguistic features of stimuli delineating their semantic category, word class, length and complexity; (2) types of cues, and their hierarchy and schedule for delivery; and (3) analysis of elicited responses, particularly the incorrect ones, for their shared attributes with the target. This intervention approach was first introduced in Western Europe in the 1970s, and it has been popular since the proliferation of research on linguistic analyses of aphasic speech. Its application is described in Shewan and Bandur's (1986) text on *Language-Oriented Approach.*

The neurolinguistic approach has tangible properties whose efficacy can be readily determined at periodic intervals. It permits evaluation and adjustment of each component of treatment (stimuli, cues and responses) and allows the client and clinician the opportunity to negotiate and refine the intervention program. An elaboration of the principles of this approach is also reflected in the section on "Treatment Parameters" in this chapter.

Pragmatic Approach

A prominent feature of this approach is that it makes a distinction between communication and language performance. Accordingly, effective communication results from successful delivery and understanding of a message, which is possible through use of appropriate pragmatic functions; conversely, it de-emphasizes use of prescriptive operant formats describing specific language modalities and linguistic parameters. In brief, it pays close attention to "what" message is communicated rather than "how" it is delivered. This approach is generally applied in socialization or group activities where the focus is on pragmatic skills that enhance conversational involvement; some examples of observed pragmatic functions include topic initiation, turn taking, elaboration or topic maintenance, content repair and clarification, and quality of listening and presupposition. A unique contribution of the pragmatic approach is its encouragement of client initiated (or preferred) method for communication wherein the client has the prerogative to select verbal and/or nonverbal mode for communication, and self-employ any inter- or intrasystemic strategy during conversational interactions. It accepts the use of nonverbal communication methods so long as they successfully communicate the message; some examples of acceptable options include use of jargon combined with appropriate speech intonation, facial expression, eye contact and hand gestures. One application of this approach is the "Promoting Aphasic Communicative Effectiveness" described by Davis (2000).

Cognitive Neuropsychological Approach

The underlying premise of this approach is to strive for "normal" or prebrain damaged performance; thus, it uses normative data as reference for establishing treatment goals. Fundamentally, this approach directs attention to treating impaired lower and higher order cognitive skills, including executive functions, and reading and writing impairments. The principles of this approach are discussed when planning intervention for cognitive-communication disorders resulting from TBI or RHI; however, it remains elusive in its elaboration.

Labels such as cognitive retraining, cognitive rehabilitation, cognitive therapy, cognitive remediation, and neurotraining have been used in reference to related intervention. Speech-language pathologists have been led to think that "cognition" is the "thinking" underlying complex language tasks requiring memory, problem solving, etc., and therefore, any intervention with the term "cognitive" is beyond the scope of their clinical practice. Esoteric labels revolving around cognition do not necessarily refer to "higher cortical functions" and any communication-related task can be argued for cognitive retraining. For example, although a simple task such as word repetition drill involves the cognitive function of STM, it is primarily a speech production task that can help reduce the symptoms of anomia or verbal apraxia.

TREATMENT PARAMETERS

The essence of treatment planning is to integrate information from factors such as individual preferences, interests, occupation, education and other personal history that can achieve successful outcome and recovery of communicative functions. Each treatment program defines appropriate objectives and describes respective procedures; these two variables and their respective components are elaborated in this section, and they are also highlighted in Figure 9.1.

Treatment objectives relate to determining the symptoms or behaviors that need to be modified, or "what" function needs to be improved. Treatment objectives are initially identified immediately following the assessment, and they are later refined and modified at different stages of intervention. Test results determine the number and type of impaired functions, while the neurological data on site and size of lesion verify the prevailing symptoms and direct attention to appropriate intra- or intersystemic reorganization strategies for intervention. Treatment objectives may be comprehensive enough to embrace multiple functions (e.g., improve functional communication), or they may be tailored to address specific symptoms (e.g., anomia, agrammatism). Comprehensive treatment programs are employed with both aphasia and cognitive communication disorders, and at all stages of recovery. Symptom-specific programs provide concentrated focus on select communication or cognitive function(s), and they are generally used during advanced stages of recovery. Irrespective of their focus, treatment objectives should delineate specific steps toward achieving communicative independence that can be expected **outside** structured treatment sessions (e.g., communicate basic physical, emotional and self-care needs, or engage in communicative interactions with family and associates).

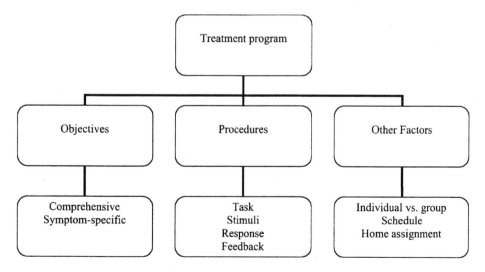

Figure 9.1. Different parameters for behavioral intervention.

Treatment procedures describe "how" the objective is to be executed during therapy, and they are explicit in describing four components: tasks (or activities), stimuli, responses, and feedback. Selection of tasks and stimuli are directly dependent on treatment objectives and they aim to alleviate or minimize the impaired symptoms. Regarding **tasks**, issues such as number of tasks that are essential for each objective, relative hierarchy and association between different tasks within an objective, and their ultimate relationship to functional communication, should be considered. The linguistic parameter of pragmatics also plays a dominant role in establishing clinician-client roles in treatment activities. Several resource materials and workbooks are available to develop tasks that are appropriate for different objectives. Typically, task presentations proceed from familiar, and less difficult, to more difficult activities; the time spent on each task should be regulated to prevent the onset of adverse behaviors.

Stimuli for a task are selected for their perceptual and linguistic attributes, their meaningfulness or importance to the individual (familiarity and frequency of use), and for their length and complexity. Perceptual components of stimuli involve manner of presentation during their input (e.g., monitoring clinician's rate, stress and inflection, and loudness for auditory presentation), and their impact on underlying cognitive functions of attention, discrimination, comprehension, retention and recall; each of these factors contribute to the quality of elicited responses. The four linguistic parameters also play an important role when selecting the stimuli and cues/strategies. For example, stimulus words representing specific word categories that are also controlled for their familiarity to the participant pertain to the semantic parameter, and those manipulated for factors such word length (number of syllables) and phonetic complexity involves the phonological parameter; at the sentence level, the morphosyntactic parameter is considered in the type of sentence structures that are used as stimuli. Of equal importance is to plan for a sufficient number of items (or trials) in a task because this factor should enforce adequate redundancy to contribute toward retention and learning; it also empowers the participant to feel the sense of accomplishment and reinforcement during the retraining. Stimuli may be selected from published word books, mass media publications, and clinical resource materials. A tenuous balance exists between stimuli and corresponding task because they contribute to the amount of time spent per task; generally, a 15–20 minute period is sufficient time for devoting intense attention to a single activity.

A **response** should be expected in some or any form but it should not to be forced. Each elicited response is generally coded for its *accuracy* (or correctness) if it meets a pre-determined target criterion. The coding system may utilize a simple bipolar (+/-) assignment, or it may be graded according to different levels (correct, cued correct, incorrect, etc); sometimes qualitative determinations are used to characterize the responses particularly those that are incorrect (e.g., types of paraphasia). Responses can also be coded for *response time* (or *latency*), which is the time interval between the presentation of a stimulus and the production of some response. Coding for response time is considered a more sensitive index because it can help make inferences regarding changes in internal neural processing from subtle temporal changes in overt performances. The distinction between response accuracy and time is frequently observed in the normal elderly and in individuals with Broca's aphasia who may indeed provide an accurate response but may do so after an abnormally long pause. Every attempt should be made to handle inaccurate or unacceptable responses otherwise the scope of intervention is violated; usually, predetermined facilitative and compensatory strategies are used to modify the inaccurate responses. Some other suggestions for improving the quality and quantity of responses include refraining from overcorrection, encouraging self-correction, providing adequate attempts and revision opportunities, and discarding a consistently difficult stimulus.

Feedback is an obligatory component of any behavioral intervention. Traditionally known as biofeedback, this concept was originally used in rehabilitation to help improve muscle performance in therapy. The contemporary term, *neurobiofeedback,* highlights the focus on improving attention, reducing anxiety and frustration, and fostering relaxation during all communicative activities. Feedback, or reinforcement, is delivered after each response either verbally or nonverbally; and it may be positive or negative in nature provided it is delivered (or received) promptly and consistently, and is directly related to the anticipated response. This treatment phase also includes provision of cues and strategies in the event of an incorrect or unacceptable response.

Each of the factors contributing to treatment delivery also requires parallel consideration of other dimensions. One of the clinical challenges includes managing and preventing the occurrences of behavioral symptoms (frustration catastrophic reaction, etc.), as well as handling interference from prevailing sensory, perceptual and motor problems. A list of some suggestions for preventing or exacerbating such inappropriate behaviors is provided in Appendix A. The forum for treatment delivery, individual versus group or specific (structured) versus nonspecific therapy, number of sessions per week, as well as duration of each session and of the entire treatment program is another equally important consideration. An efficacious treatment regimen always incorporates regular homework assignments as adjuncts to direct therapy to expedite the process of neural reorganization and retraining; the instructions for such activities should always be provided in a recorded (taped) or written format to prevent unnecessary failures and frustrations. Finally, it is always helpful to periodically audiotape or videotape a session for clinician review and self-assessment.

GROUP THERAPY

The common form of service delivery is through individualized, structured therapy. Group therapy for individuals with acquired communication disorders is frequency used as an adjunct to individual therapy, but sometimes it is used as the only form of intervention for chronic patients. The purpose of the group is to allow participants to practice identified skills and habituate strategy use; it also provides an ideal context for socialization. The ultimate goal is to generalize the relearned skills in social interactions. Social adjustment problems with family and associates occur as a consequence of brain damage and they may not decease without corrective measures; inappropriate social behaviors can lead to loss of employment, and a life of isolation and loneliness because of interpersonal difficulties.

Communication-oriented goals in group therapy relate to sharpening pragmatic and social skills during group discourse in a less structured, but more challenging environment than can be provided in one-on-one treatment sessions. Specific objectives for group members are established from identified deficit areas; some examples include word retrieval, verbal organization, or interpretation of verbal and nonverbal messages. The clinician may provide the stimuli and feedback at the onset of a new task, with the responsibility of providing feedback gradually transitioned to group members. The ultimate goal is to foster independence and therefore, clinician modeling and assistance is incorporated only as needed.

Group activities may include discussion of a theme or topic, debates and role plays. They may also address goals pertaining to giving and receiving feedback in a noncritical manner, higher-level verbal organization, speed of processing information, and listening skills. The format may involve members choosing a topic among themselves and then break into teams. Selection of problematic topics is appropriate for group activities, and they may include dealing with uncomfortable or difficult questions, discussing their medical problems, forgetting names of familiar and important people in their lives, and how to seek assistance from strangers in a difficult or unfamiliar situation.

Strategies that may be helpful during group activities include brainstorming, outlining and note taking. The underlying premise is to promote a sense of ownership, collaboration and practice. Entering a conversation is difficult for most individuals but more so for individuals with communication disorders due to their impaired comprehension of overall or subtle nuances of conveyed message, processing multiple pieces of information, and difficulty with self-expression. Some strategies for self-expression in challenging situations include developing a list of appropriate entrance phrases, identifying main point and follow it with details (thought sequencing), and practicing preferred nonverbal strategies.

Time limits should be established for topic preparation and presentation. Group peers can be directed to review fellow members' performances for presence or absence of select communication behaviors during the activity. For example, they may evaluate for factors such as word choice, tone of voice, appropriateness and amount of verbal output, effective use of speaking time, organization of the presentation, providing constructive input, handling feedback from colleagues, and effective use of learned strategies.

In addition to improvement in communication, there are other psychosocial benefits of group intervention:

- *Ventilation:* the process of talking about one's problems with peers tends to reduce the tension with family and associates.
- *Reassurance:* the realization that other people have encountered similar problems and obstacles, and they have handled them as well.

- *Education:* teaching and learning with peers reduces the level of anxiety by removing doubts and confusion about the disorder and related symptoms.
- *Kinship:* sharing responsibility develops relationships, collegiality, and also helps reduce anxiety by turning to others for advice.
- *Optimism:* adopting a constructive outlook by stressing the positive aspects and outlooks of rehabilitation helps develop a sense of confidence with the new self-image.

Thus conversational groups provide a safe arena for practicing learned skills, and gaining the confidence to return to their social settings and community.

MANAGEMENT STRATEGIES FOR DEMENTIA

The role of the speech-language pathologist is to assist in the diagnostic process and in the management of available communication competency at different stages of dementia. The management process involves making periodic adjustments to the communication environment to help sustain some degree of interaction between the individual and respective caregivers. Unlike other diagnostic categories, the focus is on maintenance of preserved symptoms, and thus management goals for dementia are palliative in nature.

In addition to the list of suggestions in Appendix A, the following considerations help enhance communication of individuals with dementia:

- control the environmental stimuli by assuring that memorable objects that are important to the individual are placed in a consistent location in their personal space;
- engage the individual in group socialization activities utilizing multimodal stimulation with emphasis on consistent and intensified use of visual modality;
- determine the optimal type and number of conversational partners; generally, same (familiar) individuals and fewer participants enhance interaction behaviors;
- employ external (visual) memory aids in the form of personal photo albums and scrap books as stimuli for conversation topics to promote attention and interaction;
- attend to concurrent sensory (hearing and visual) problems because

they may exacerbate problem behaviors; for example, repetition of the same questions, increased arguments and restlessness may be related to confusion created by faulty hearing which can be addressed with contemporary hearing aids that require minimal client collaboration.

A couple behavioral intervention strategies have shown successful results for individuals with dementia. One of these is *priming,* which involves developing a connection (association) between two consecutive, related stimuli to maintain attention and facilitate a response; thus priming is another form of intrasystemic association strategy. Another technique, *spaced retrieval,* requires repeated recall of target concepts (name or event) at increasingly longer intervals of time and with intervening tasks and distractions. This strategy for memory intervention was first described by Landauer and Bjork (1978), and it has shown beneficial outcome on retention of learned/trained information in individuals with dementia as well.

TREATMENT EFFICACY

The brain's plasticity is the primary reason for not giving up on any individual. However, the effectiveness of any treatment has to be justified, and in this instance it relates to language rehabilitation. Treatment efficacy relates to *accountability,* or appropriateness and quality of delivered therapy, which is a paramount consideration of patients and their families, as well as reimbursement agencies; each of these parties seek indicators that the delivered treatment can yield successful outcome. Budgetary issues have resulted in reduction of rehabilitation programs however, the myriad needs of the neurologically-damaged individual persists. Funding agencies such as insurance companies and state vocational rehabilitation agencies mandate that all therapies relate specifically to outcome goals that strive for some level of employment or pre-morbid communication functions; these criteria direct attention to *efficiency* of rendered services, which enables financial sponsors to place arbitrary limitations to contain treatment costs. Thus the issue of treatment efficacy addresses both clinical accountability and efficiency to demonstrate the benefits of the intervention to the patient. The contemporary notion of *evidence-based practice* is a derivative of this issue but it is not as all encompassing as the concept of treatment efficacy. This section introduces some indicators describing clinical practice issues that relate to treatment efficacy for adults with aphasia and cognitive-communication disorders.

Assessment Protocol

An informed and knowledgeable clinician always utilizes a standard assessment protocol. Use of functional communication protocols and subjective methods, and caregiver and family member's reports, can serve as estimates for determining progress; however, sole reliance on this form of diagnostic process can lead to false positive or negative impressions regarding a patient's communication performance. Casual observations of care givers may also misrepresent the type and severity of the communication problem and also provide unreliable information. Such methods for data collection in clinical practice may adversely impact clinician reputation and reimbursement of rendered services as well.

Type of Treatment

The clinician who is knowledgeable of different treatment approaches and related methods, and utilizes them to meet each patient's unique needs is both accountable and efficient in service delivery. This competency is achieved through an understanding of evidence-based literature on treatment options for different linguistic-communication symptom; this knowledge provides the basis for selecting appropriate goals and strategies for different disorders. Such self-study habits can also guide a resourceful clinician to defy common misconceptions and stereotypes regarding select disorders. One illustration in point is the presumption that individuals with global aphasia do not generally improve from speech-language therapy; careful review of related research however, has clearly identified two issues, assessment method (caregiver perceptions versus standardized test results) and type of treatment (generic programmed instruction versus neurolinguistic approach), that explain the misinformation (Sarno, Silverman & Sands, 1970; Sarno & Levita, 1971; Sarno & Levita, 1981).

A speech-language pathologist should not be offended if the client seeks verification of clinical expertise in neurogenic communication disorders; this is analogous to seeking similar assurance from a cardiologist who diagnoses and determines the candidacy for a coronary by-pass surgery. An obvious indicator of clinician incompetency is the regular use of a rigid programmed approach (or canned treatment protocol) for each of the referred patients irrespective of the severity and nature of the communication problem. The clinician should be familiar with field tested treatment methods for different language related symptoms; this understanding is substantiated in reported significant improvements in auditory and verbal modalities irrespective of type and severity of aphasia (Basso, Capitani & Vignolo, 1979). Another example is the proven efficiency of the Melodic Intonation Therapy and use of music for nonfluent patients and those with Broca's aphasia (Helm-Estabrooks & Albert, 2004; Luria, 1980).

Type of Disorder

Regarding aphasia, there is sufficient evidence affirming that individuals with Broca's and anomic aphasia benefit from treatment. This finding is true even when these groups of individuals receive the intervention following the period of spontaneous (physiological) recovery provided treatment objectives focused on their primary symptoms (Brindley, Copeland, Demain & Martyn, 1989). There is ample evidence supporting positive outcome for individuals with TBI (Coelho, DeRuyter & Stein, 1996). Also, some favorable documentation is available regarding recovery from intervention for individuals with language of confusion (Drummond, 1986).

Prognostic Variables

The clinician must have a firm understanding of the different positive and negative prognostic factors that apply to each individual and weigh them carefully to make a summative judgment regarding their cumulative contribution to rehabilitation goals and outcome. Each of the different possible variables are described as reference in Chapter 8.

Clinician Competency

This attribute is reflected in the ability to formulate appropriate clinical impressions, recommendations and their justifications based on professional experiences and documentation of previous cases with similar problems. This competency is acquired through related diagnostic and intervention experiences and utilization of necessary critical thinking skills in regards to all clinical situations. In addition, professional practice habits relating to maintaining precise internal records on treatment objectives with corresponding procedures and anticipated responses, their periodic assessment and review, and incorporating contributing background information (age, etiology, medical and personal history) are of equal importance; such thorough recordkeeping pattern also enables the clinician to confidently discuss elicited responses according to rate and pattern of recovery for select symptoms and disorders.

Manner of Service Delivery

Selection and documentation of type, number and duration of treatment sessions for the different disorders is crucial for demonstrating accountability and efficiency for reimbursement of rendered services. There is sufficient evidence in support of individualized, symptom-specific intervention. Also, there is some data attesting that individuals who receive therapy administered by a speech-language pathologist show greater improvement than those receiving therapy delivered by nursing staff (Shewan & Kertesz, 1984). The importance of having a qualified clinician deliver the necessary services is confirmed irrespective of the location where therapy is delivered (clinic or home). The data on individual versus group therapy are paradoxical due to confounding effects of variables relating to differences in types of assessment and treatment methodologies for each of these forms of therapy (Wertz et al., 1981).

Onset of Therapy

The largest historical evidence has established that earlier the initiation of therapy the greater and quicker is the recovery (Wylie, 1970). Although this finding is based on the benefits of maximal possible improvement during the period of spontaneous recovery, there is sufficient evidence supporting the fact that individuals with non-progressive brain damage do recover beyond the spontaneous recovery period provided factors governing type of disorder and type of treatment are maintained (Basso et al., 1979; Davis, 2000; Poeck, Huber & Willmes, 1989; Sarno & Levita, 1981).

Other Treatment Variables

Factors such as rate of learning do indeed distinguish individuals with brain damage as slow learners; however the shape of their learning curve remains identical to their peers with no brain damage (Tikofsky, 1971). Also, there is sufficient evidence suggesting reduction in response latency (time) as a manifestation of recovery thus validating its use for recording subtle improvements in communication performances across all severity levels.

BIOLOGICAL EVIDENCE

Studies of mammals and nonmammals conducted in the 1990s have shown positive benefits of training and rehabilitation. For example, bees learn to differentiate flowers with good nectar from those with bitter (or poisonous) nectar but they learn to do so at different rates based on age (or experience) and level of motivation. Corroboration can also be found from canary birds who show that those exposed to tape recordings of canary songs (or "stimulated") revealed 10 times greater amount of RNA at autopsy than those who were not exposed to similar stimulation. Finally, studies on stimulation of older rodents show that they learned new information just as well as their younger counterparts.

In humans, it seems that learning, exercise and environmental stimulation result in increase in neurotransmitters, neuronal activity and synapses; they also stimulate neurogenesis in the hippocampus. These occurrences are explained through the concept of *long-term synaptic potentiation (LTP)*, which involves establishment of synapses resulting from repeated stimulations of a neural circuitry. The increase in synaptic efficacy result as a consequence of molecular (positive) changes in calcium and glutamate, and it is observed in the hippocampus (Kiernan, 2005). Macroscopically, LTP is used to explain the formation of long-term memories, and it justifies the use of multiple trials (or repetitions) of the same activity during treatment delivery. Pavlovian dog experiments have inspired us to theorize that learning is enhanced when one makes association (connection) between a stimulus and its consequence. This is the basis for forming cellular circuits and ultimately learning and retraining of adults with brain damage.

OTHER CONSIDERATIONS

One of the primary goals for a person with brain damage is to resume their routine lives at home and at work. While much of the responsibility to return to normal life falls on individual patients, their families, friends, employers and co-workers serve as key members at different stages of recovery; these associates provide the necessary support, empathy, and practical assistance to help the person in the adjustment process. Sometimes these caring individuals tend to understand physiological injuries better than cognitive-communication impairments because these deficits may not be as evident. Increasing their sensitivity to factors such as experiencing fatigue, requiring additional time to complete a task, difficulty following multistep instructions, refraining from casual conversations in noisy environments, avoiding telephone conversations, and withdrawal from exuberant social activities may preserve and enhance their social ties and commitments. Therefore, it is important to attempt to change the communicative styles of caregivers via counseling and modeling techniques. An understanding of each of these issues may promote fruitful relationships and prevent further emotional and psychological problems for any individual member. Some positive outcomes may be acceptance of a part-time job if full-time employment is not possible, learning new skills, and focus on the "abilities" rather than the disabilities.

SUMMARY

The scope of linguistic-communication therapy is to determine the nature of the deficits, ascertain their impact on routine interaction, and attempt to remediate the deficits via facilitating toward "normalcy" or compensate for the deficits by enhancing other avenues for communication. In case of progressive or severe cognitive-communication disorders a realistic goal is to increase opportunities for communication via socialization and group therapy. Each of these targets is approached via direct intervention approaches.

During the acute stages of hospitalization, one "manages" the prevailing disorder by conducting *diagnostic therapy* which is composed of parallel consideration of stabilizing observed symptoms, providing specific or nonspecific stimulation to improve performance, and educating and counseling the individual and caregiver(s) regarding the symptoms and management/rehabilitation goals. As the individual stabilizes, or at various intervals during chronic stages, there is greater emphasis on treatment of impaired symptoms and rehabilitation outcome. Along this continuum, referral and discharge decisions need to be negotiated upon consideration of several factors including extent of prevailing symptoms, trend of progress/recovery, the individual's motivation and attitude toward therapy, and financial issues pertaining to insurance and reimbursement. Although treatment termination is a reality, it is important to have the patients' best interest in mind when making such a decision.

The benefits of an intervention depend on four considerations: treatment approach and planning, manner of treatment delivery, and lots of practice opportunities. Each of these factors increase sensory input and motor functions which in turn result in LTP and epitomize brain plasticity, and are overtly reflected as improvement of functions. A competent clinician is able to integrate different treatment philosophies to create unique intervention approach that is most appropriate for the individual and thus achieve maximum reorganization of functions. Based on my clinical experiences, I strongly believe that 90 percent of successful outcome of intervention that occurs following the physiological (spontaneous) recovery is to be credited to the delivering clinician.

Appendix A

GENERAL SUGGESTIONS FOR COMMUNICATING WITH ELDERS

Approach the individual from the front so they are not startled.

Identify or introduce yourself, and establish eye contact before speaking.

Sit at the individual's eye level to promote visual stimulation and to help adjust for any hearing loss.

Dress conservatively, and wear bright colors to help promote attention and conversation.

Address the person by his/her name (get name during the introduction or from the staff).

Select familiar topics that pertain to the present (event, environment, weather, holiday, pet), and maintain focus on the positive aspects of life or their condition.

Speak clearly and slowly in simple and direct statements during all interactions, and repeat important information; use nonverbal cues (picture, writing, gesture) to supplement verbal interactions.

Refrain from being too friendly or too distant, and from assuming an authoritative role or speaking in childish/patronizing manner.

Assume the primary role of a listener by posing open-ended questions, pretending to be less knowledgeable of the topic, and refrain from discussing personal experiences and preferences.

Encourage some response even if it is in the form of direct eye contact, but refrain from enforcing a response.

Allow the individual to initiate tactile contact but the clinician may only do so with caution in case of an aversive reaction.

Permit the individual to "communicate" even if the response is inaccurate or irrelevant; provide adequate response time, and monitor interruptions and overcorrections.

198

Avoid provision of details or overelaboration of the same subject, and refrain from use of professional jargon.

Encourage self-evaluation of performances and improvement.

Recognize and empathize with the individual regarding their frustrations during communication.

Use explicit preparatory phrases to introduce ("I want you to") and terminate topics ("Do you have any questions?" or "Now, we will try another activity").

Always terminate the interaction or session with a departing signal.

Utilize distractions to divert an agitated individual's attention.

Chapter 10

OTHER INTERVENTION APPROACHES

Individuals with brain damage receive several forms of intervention. Typically, medical (or pharmacological) management is the treatment of choice obviously because patients are seen first by the primary care provider (physician) who responds to the patient's need for a quick resolution to the problem. Surgical intervention is another invasive option that is employed less often and tends to be dependent on select diagnosis. Other esoteric forms of treatments have also been mentioned in related literature and they also have implications for neurogenic communication disorders. Finally, management areas targeting quality of life issues for the brain-damaged individual are also considered in an optimal and comprehensive rehabilitation program. The ideal aspiration is to strive for 100 percent repair, or ultimate healing, of the damaged tissue using all possible options. This mission is reflected in contemporary utilization of a variety of concurrent treatments involving both physicians and rehabilitation professionals; therefore, information regarding some medical, surgical, and other forms of interventions for adults with neurogenic communication disorders is introduced in this chapter.

PHARMACOLOGICAL INTERVENTION

Pharmacological management of adults involves use of prescription drugs which can be organized into two major categories: preventive and symptomatic drugs. Preventive drugs are generally prescribed to individuals who may be at risk for developing a brain damage. Other drugs are prescribed to minimize or alleviate the effects (symptoms) of the impaired neural mechanism. Each of these groups of pharmacotherapies is described in this section, and they are also listed in Table 10.1.

Preventive Drugs

The underlying premise of preventive medication is to help an individual circumvent or at least postpone becoming a victim of brain damage. One example is prescribing select drugs to individuals with the diagnosis of arteriosclerosis with the objective of preventing the possibility of incurring an occlusive CVA. A common prescription for such cases is the use of *anticoagulants* (*platelet antiaggregants* or blood thinners) to help prevent the risk of clot formation; an example is the benefit from daily low dose intake of aspirin in men. Regular use of aspirin and other nonsteroidal *antiinflammatory* drugs have also been found to reduce the risk of developing symptoms of dementia. Other drugs that can contribute to lowering the risk of CVA include: cholesterol reducing drugs aimed to retard arterial plaque deposition; *antihypertensives* (and angiotension-converting enzyme inhibitors) help dilate blood vessels to lower blood pressure and improve vascular efficiency; *antidiabetics* (insulin therapy) to regulate insulin levels in type I and II diabetes; and *diuretics* to lower cellular and bodily fluid regulation by increasing the volume of urine and salt released by the kidneys. Most often diuretics are used to treat hypertension and congestive heart disease, but they can also serve to lower intracranial CSF pressure as a symptomatic therapy.

Symptomatic Drugs

Aggressive pharmacological intervention is implemented when a person shows signs of brain dysfunction or following a positive diagnosis of brain pathology. The resultant myriad symptoms, and contributing conditions, call for administering several different types of drugs and consequently, symptomatic drugs are further organized according to three subcategories. One of these categories directly targets the damaged vascular (circulatory) system. A common option is the administration of *thrombolytic* (clot dissolving) agents which are a special type of anticoagulants given within the first few (3) hours **after** the onset of an ischemic (occlusive) CVA. The most popular thrombolytic agent, *tissue Plasmogen Activator* (tPA), is administered intra-

Table 10.1. Different Types of Pharmocological Interventions.

Preventive drugs	Vascular	Symptomatic drugs Psychotropic	Neurotropic
Anticoagulants	Thromolytics	Antidepressants	Pain killers
Antinflammatory	Diuretics	Anxiolytes	Anticonvulsants
Cholesterol reducers			Memory enhancers
Antihypertensives			Neurostimulants
Antidiabetics			
Diuretics			

venously to individuals with ischemic CVA after ruling out the presence of cerebral hematoma or hemorrhage from a CT scan. The outcome of administering tPA has been positive in terms of minimizing, and even eliminating symptoms in the majority of individuals with the CVA; in a small percentage (3–6%) of individuals however, tPA can increase the risk of intracranial hemorrhage and may cause another CVA. Other clot-dissolving agents have also been introduced as alternatives to tPA for individuals who do not meet the narrow window of time required for tPA administration. Sometimes corticosteroids and osmotic diuretics are used to reduce cerebral edema, and thus reduce intracranial CSF pressure to help restore cerebral circulation (see Table 10.1).

The other two categories of symptomatic medications directly influence neuronal and synaptic activities. Of these, *psychotropic drugs* strive to regulate mood and behavioral anomalies. Drugs classified as antipsychotic (or neuroleptic) agents that are delivered to treat psychiatric symptoms such as hallucinations and delusions are excluded from this discussion to maintain focus on the content of the text. A commonly prescribed psychotropic group of drugs are *antidepressants,* which serve to alleviate symptoms of depression in normal and brain-damaged adults; these drugs can enhance social interaction and motivation for communication. Although adverse reactions of antidepressants have not been documented among elderly adults, their use has been linked with suicidal and violent behaviors in teenaged children, some of who may have a history of head trauma as well. Antianxiety agents or *anxiolytes* (sedatives and tranquilizers) represent the class of psychotropic drugs that help induce relaxation and reduce tension (stress); these drugs may range from relatively tame, common sedatives to include drugs that have more potent effects on brain activity (see Table 10.1).

The last category of symptomatic drugs, *neurotropic drugs,* aims to modify the neurological symptoms and thus improve disrupted functions. One group, *anticonvulsants* (or antiseizure medication), is commonly prescribed for individuals with idiopathic epilepsy to control the onset and intensity of the seizures. Anticonvulsants are also administered to acute brain-damaged patients to prevent aversive electrical activity during the early days of brain reorganization. Another class of neuroleptics is *nootropic drugs* that help enhance memory and attention. These drugs are increasingly prescribed to arrest or slow down the progression of mild-moderate symptoms of dementia. Some of these drugs, grouped as cholinesterase inhibitors (or anticholinesterase drugs) help stop breakdown of acetylcholine and improve cholinergic function (inhibit acetylcholinesterase); they also accelerate neural conduction and cause synapses to remain open for a fractional longer second to boost the flow of glutamate. Overtly, these drugs help improve alertness, routine everyday functions, recalling ability and other cognitive functions. It is important to caution that memory enhancing drugs do not cure or reverse the dementia. Another class of drugs grouped as *neurostimulants* have shown mixed results. Traditional studies of Bromocriptine® (a dopamine agonist) as a stimulant for individuals with head injury have failed to demonstrate positive effects. However, use of derivatives of amphetamine has shown to improve communication and cognitive performances. Finally, recent developments have shown that some drugs can stimulate premature (stem) cells to multiply and mature into the cells responsible for memory functions; the outcome of such investigations show promising future for restoring cognitive mechanisms involved in learning and memory (see Table 10.1).

The field of pharmacology studies the interaction between a drug and a living system. It reports beneficial results of drugs on the targeted symptoms and cautions against their adverse effects on metabolic functions of other organs involved with the gastrointestinal and cardiovascular systems. Pharmacology also provokes issues pertaining to rate and extent of absorption of prescriptive drugs, and the relationship between age and body mass on the distribution and metabolism of different drugs. The popularity of pharmacotherapy is daunting because it tends to side step issues regarding drug habituation and abuse, and their long-term effects on neuronal metabolism and functions. Finally, it needs to be noted that the presented information on symptomatic drugs has focused exclusively on "synthetic" drugs developed in laboratory conditions and manufactured by pharmaceutical companies. There is emerging evidence on use of natural (herbal) remedies for alleviating pain, and for inducing brain stimulation and relaxation. For example, extracts of leaves of Gingko biloba tree has shown beneficial effects as an anticoagulant and as a memory enhancer. Perhaps there is promising future for incorporating such alternative remedies for neurological disorders.

SURGICAL INTERVENTION

Several forms of surgical management have been developed for the different neuropathologies of the brain (see Table 10.2). Some of these methods are directed toward occlusive CVAs particularly for arteriosclerotic and thrombotic CVAs. A brief description of these options is provided in this section:

- *Carotid endarterectomy* is one of the traditional approaches and precursor to contemporary options. This procedure involves reopening the arteriosclerotic vessel to remove the plaque. Later modifications aimed to minimize the risk for an embolism (or embolic CVA) by employing laser technology to raise tissue temperature at wavelengths that are sufficient to help absorb the arteriosclerotic plaque.

- *Extracranial-to-Intracranial Anastomosis (ECIC)* is a traditional "by-pass" procedure where a branch of a healthy artery is attached above an arteriosclerotic vessel to by-pass the stenotic (occluded) region of an artery. For example, a smaller branch of the healthy external carotid artery, such as the superficial temporal or occipital artery, may serve as the donor vessel to be surgically connected to a cortical branch of the middle cerebral artery in the presence of an occluded internal carotid artery; in this instance the internal carotid artery is by-passed by the donor artery. The

ECIC procedure requires a minimum 2 millimeter diameter blood vessel for the donor artery.

- *Balloon angioplasty,* another option for removal of the arteriosclerotic plaque, utilizes a balloon tip catheter that is inserted into the artery to reach the target location. The tiny balloon at the tip of the catheter is inflated to stretch the plaque-filled stenotic artery and cause the plaque to split up. The possibility of an embolism as a complication, and the tendency for reclosing the clogged artery, serve to reduce the benefits of this procedure. A recent variation uses a balloon guide catheter encasing a 1.1 millimeter wide flexible microcatheter (corkscrew-like metal wire) that is guided into the femoral artery (in groin area) to snake its way to reach the carotid artery and the region of the clot. The wire ensnares the clot and pulls it out while the external ballooned tube is kept inflated to widen and slow the blood flow within the artery (Merci Retrieval System, 2005).

Some surgical options for nonocclusive CVAs such as aneurysm and AVM have also been described in the literature (see Table 10.2). Of these a couple of approaches aim to prevent the possibility of a hemorrhage in individuals with cerebral aneurysm:

- *Clipping* the aneurysm involves placement of a reinforcement, or "clip" on the weakened arterial wall to prevent the possibility of a rupture and thus prevent a hemorrhage.
- *Embolotherapy* (or *embolization*) utilizes the principle of balloon angioplasty, and it is used for both aneurysm and AVM. A tiny detachable pellet (silicon or glue-like substance), placed at the tip of a thin catheter is inserted via the carotid artery to plug the aneurysm; the pellet can also seal off some of the tangled vessels in AVM and thus prevent the backflow of deoxygenated blood. In cases of head injury where there is CSF leak due to a fractured ethmoid (cranial bone), the leak is plugged with the help of an endoscope directed via the nose and some "glue" (sometimes patient's blood) used to secure the plug.
- *Stereotactic radiotherapy* (*Proton therapy* or *gamma knife surgery*) involves the delivery of high doses of accurately targeted radiation to "noninvasively" ablate some blood vessels in AVM or destroy brain tumors. The "stereotactic" component of the procedure utilizes a metal frame that is bolted to the skull to stabilize the head and obtain a precise marking of the target (tumor or

Table 10.2. Surgical Options for the Different Neuropathologies.

Options	Arteriosclerosis	Thrombosis	Aneurysm	Arteriovenous malformation	Head injury	Tumor	Other etiologies
Carotid endarterectomy	Yes	Yes	–	–	–	–	–
Extra-Intracranial Anastomosis	Yes	–	–	–	–	–	–
Balloon angioplasty	Yes	Yes	Yes	Yes	–	–	–
Clipping of artery–	–	–	Yes	–	–	–	–
Embolotherapy	–	–	Yes	Yes	Yes	–	–
Stereotactic radiotherapy	–	–	–	Yes	–	Yes	–
CSF shunting	–	–	–	–	Yes	–	NPH*
Cerebral disconnection	–	–	–	–	–	–	Epilepsy
Hemispherectomy	–	–	–	–	–	Yes	Epilepsy

*Normal Pressure Hydrocephalus

AVM) location. Next, the radiation therapy is delivered to the target site; this procedure allows reaching difficult areas particularly those in the deep regions and is therefore, considered less traumatic to the adjacent healthy tissue. Radiation therapy destroys the tumerous tissue; in case of AVM, it is also applied to select blood vessels to seal off the lumen so the singed vessel serves as obstruction to prevent the backflow of deoxygenated blood.

The surgical procedure of *CSF shunting* is used to lower and monitor CSF pressure in individuals immediately following a TBI. Usually a *burr hole* is made with a special ("burr") drill bit to penetrate through the skull and the subarachnoid space; a bolt is placed here to monitor the CSF flow in the presence of increased intracranial pressure. CSF shunting is also beneficial for stabilizing and even improving cognitive functions in individuals diagnosed with Normal Pressure Hydrocephalus and those with Alzheimer's disease. In such instances, the process is a little different; the shunt system is implanted permanently (under the skin), and it consists of three components:

1. collection catheter situated within the cerebral ventricles or the lumbar spinal canal;
2. differential pressure valve to regulate CSF flow; and
3. drainage catheter to channel the CSF away from the brain to either the peritoneal cavity (*ventriculoperitoneal/lumboperitoneal shunt*) or the carotid vein (*ventriculoatrial shunt*) where it can be absorbed.

Some adverse effects of shunt implantation may be "siphoning" out of excessive CSF resulting in headache and nausea in the upright position; in some instances, subdural hematoma may result as a complication as well.

Occasionally, surgical management is considered as the last option for children with severe epilepsy who do not benefit from the preferred anticonvulsant drugs. The surgery involves either destruction (ablation) or removal of neural tissue through a variety of procedures; the goal is to prevent the spread of seizure activity from the pathological area to healthier parts of the brain. One option is *cerebral disconnection,* or *split-brain surgery,* which involves disconnecting the interconnecting white matter between the two hemispheres; the severation may entail the corpus callosum or *callosectomy,* or the anterior commissure (*commissurotomy*).

Another surgical option is *hemispherectomy,* which entails removal of a large amount of neural tissue within a hemisphere. This is a much drastic option for children with severe epilepsy (Rasmusen's encephalopathy) and in those with brain tumors. In general, the region that triggers the seizures, or the cancerous tissue, is excised. Although the consequence of such surgery is ominous, it is selected as the last recourse to offer relief from the seizures in children and young adults, and hopefully restore some degree of quality of life. This form of management relies on the premise of *cerebral plasticity* implying that the young brain is relatively pliable, or "plastic," and therefore it will permit the residual intact areas to learn, compensate and assume functions of the removed brain tissue. There is a critical period however, beyond which either hemisphere cannot make a dramatic adjustment for loss of function; usually this period occurs sometime between the first and fifteenth birthday after which the brain is "hard wired" and tends to be relatively less adaptive to reorganization.

NEUROSTIMULATION APPROACHES

The fundamental principle of neurostimulation is to administer electrical stimulation either directly or indirectly. The direct method of delivering neurostimulation utilizes a matchbox-sized, battery-operated microprocessor that is surgically implanted into the cranium for individuals with epilepsy. Its electrodes pick up abnormal electrical impulses that signal an oncoming seizure, and deter the onset of the seizure by delivering a burst of electrical activity to the brain. This exogenous input overwhelms the internal turbulent region and resets the brain's electrical rhythm to stop the seizure. The programming of the device and placement of the electrodes is customized for each patient to gain maximal benefits; the device has a wireless connection to a laptop personal computer to make any adjustments to its programming.

Electrical stimulation can also be delivered indirectly to the brain via *Trancranial Magnetic Stimulation* (TMS). TMS is used for patients with severe depression and it has been introduced as a possible treatment option for individuals with neurological disorders as well. The procedure entails placing the TMS stimulating device against the cranium; the device generates a magnetic field via an electrical current to its wire coil. The cells in the region where the magnetic field meets the brain tissue create an electrical impulse that scrambles the surrounding neural activity, causing a kind of blackout in the target region. A series of pulses are thus transmitted, and the subject merely senses a feeling of tapping on the head caused by the contraction of the scalp muscles. The positive effect of TMS has been reported to last for a few hours following a single treatment. In animal experiments, TMS produces changes in levels of neurotransmitters and in synaptic activity, which hint at the possibility of long-term changes. This method assists in mapping the circuits of the normal brain and can reveal any faulty wiring; it has the potential to serve both diagnostic and therapeutic function. Application of TMS for neurological disorders such as Parkinson's disease have yielded questionable results, while it shows promise for use in epilepsy. Factors such as frequency, intensity and duration of stimulation, as well as number and length of treatments are not yet established for this procedure.

GENETIC ENGINEERING APPLICATIONS

This topic involves growing human nervous tissue in special medium (culture) and implantation (or grafting) of genetically modified tissue to the human body. If the target tissue relates to the nervous system then the designated term *neuroimplantation* is applicable. Some examples include implanting genetically modified cells that releases NGF into dying brain cells aiming to increase the density of neurons that support memory functions. Another form of neuroimplantation used as an experimental option for individuals with aggressive brain tumors is *virotherapy* where genetically altered (reproduced) viruses are delivered to kill the tumor cells.

Trials on chronic stroke patients have shown cautiously promising results with cell implantation. Laboratory cultured neurons from embryonic-like stem cells, culled from cancerous tumors, are injected to the target site that is identified with the assistance of a stereotactic frame and from CT or MRI scans. Comparison of PET scans taken prior to and six months following the implantation has shown greater than 10 percent increase in metabolic activity (uptake of glucose) in the damaged area; these findings have also been corroborated with positive changes in neurological examinations as well (Meltzer, Konziolka, Villemagne, Wechsler, Goldstein, Thulborn et al., 2001).

HYPERBARIC OXYGEN THERAPY

This treatment involves breathing 100 percent oxygen (O_2) while in a pressurized (hyperbaric) enclosed chamber. The underlying premise is that inhaling the pressurized O_2 supersaturates the plasma, which then oozes through stenotic blood vessels to reach the damaged area. The mitochondria in cells use the O_2 to resume their metabolic functions and thus restore the functions of the adjacent issue. Proponents of hyperbaric O_2 recommend receiving this form of treatment on a daily basis for patients with CVA; however, it has failed to show any improvement of communication functions in individuals with CVA (Sarno, Rusk, Diller & Sarno, 1972). It also needs to be noted that excessive O_2 can be toxic to normal, healthy tissue. An adaptation of this concept is use of routine hyperventilation. This format has been applied to individuals with TBI with the assumption that it keeps the patient well oxygenated, decreases arterial carbon dioxide (CO_2), and controls acidosis; however, each of these factors can contribute to secondary brain injury. Also, excessive hyperventilation can be dangerous and therefore, contraindicated for common use.

ASSISTIVE TECHNOLOGY

Hearing impairment is a common disorder among the elderly including individuals with aphasia and cognitive-communication disorders and it can exacerbate the prevailing symptoms. It is also speculated that faulty hearing may contribute to some of the overt behavioral problems as well. A valid option is to fit the individual with a *hearing aid* which serves to amplify the incoming auditory signal. Traditionally, individuals with aphasia and cognitive-communication disorders have not been considered good candidates for hearing aids because they have difficulty communicating whether or not the devices help them hear better and also because the devices require a lot of instruction in care and use. New developments in hearing aid technology have now resulted in simpler devices that minimize patient involvement and are more comfortable to wear. Hearing aids can improve the quality of the incoming auditory message, decrease the confusion experienced in communication situations, and result in fewer and less severe problem behaviors in individuals with neurogenic communication disorders.

Technologies designed to support communication in the form of *augmentative* and *alternative communication* (AAC) systems are used to enhance (augment) the individual's ability to communicate; or they can be employed to circumvent (replace) the impaired channels of communication. Such options are considered for individuals with severe communication problems who have very limited verbal output such as those with Broca's and global aphasia. Generally, AAC systems represent visual symbols in the form of written text, freehand drawing, pictures or icons, and hand/facial gestures; the goal is to help improve comprehension of the incoming message and express routine needs. The AAC systems may incorporate low or complex ("high") technologies. An AAC system is considered "low tech" if it is simple in its format and utilizes minimal to no technology (e.g., paper, pen, pictorial cards, hand gestures, and electronic typing devices). Some examples of low tech AAC options that are promoted for individuals with aphasia include generic alphabet boards, communication cards, picture books, American Indian Gestural Code or "Amerind" (Skelly, 1979), and Visual Action Therapy and drawing for communication (Helm-Estabrooks & Albert, 2004). High tech AAC systems require sophisticated and costly electronic equipment involving computers, related peripherals, and software with speech synthesizers.

Other assistive devices relate to improving limb performance; their discussion however, does not directly relate to improving communication performance and is therefore, beyond the scope of this text.

OTHER THERAPIES

The most common adjuncts to speech-language therapy are *physical* and *occupational therapies.* Any form of physical exercise improves blood flow and oxygen to the entire system including the brain where it may release select neurotransmitters to enhance arousal, attention and brain activity. Occupational therapy can reinforce communication goals by incorporating them into activities of daily living (ADL) exercises. Combining physical exercise with a patient's communication and cognitive goals provides an opportunity to be mainstreamed and feel successful; it also incorporates the principle of intersystemic reorganization. For example, rhythmic speech and motor exercises can be delivered in an interdisciplinary team environment under combined guidance of the speech-language pathologist, as well as occupational and physical therapists. The patient may call out the exercises or count the beats aloud while performing the exercises; successful completion of series of exercises also help toward improving comprehension, memory and executive function (sequential performance) problems. Each of these rehabilitation professionals can also serve as consultants regarding verification of patient compliancy and generalization of communication performance.

Lifestyle factors that influence the onset of a stroke are also important for significantly reducing the likelihood of another one. For example, the risk of stroke in people who quit smoking decreases significantly in just two years and within five years their risk of having a stroke is the same as someone who has never smoked. Similarly, other positive changes in diet and activity such as a low-fat, low-salt diet combined with limited alcohol intake and a regular exercise program can prevent a large percentage of CVAs and other diseases as well. Recent information from animal models indicates that diet rich in antioxidant vitamins, found in fruits and vegetables, has beneficial effects not only on cardiovascular functions but also serves to protect the brain by limiting the amount of damage in the event of a CVA. Therefore, *nutritional counseling* can be an integral prophylactic component since many patients also have concurrent conditions such as diabetes and cardiovascular disorders; these conditions must be controlled while the brain is healing from the damage.

All individuals flourish in a nurturing environment, and the same principle applies to individuals with neurological disorders; a popular medium to promote this ideology is through *support groups*. Community-based and institutional support groups serve an important psychosocial function for both the victims of brain damage and their respective caregivers. Each of these members can commonly benefit from participation in support groups in several ways: develop a sense of identity; gain peer support; discuss emotional needs and problems; share and develop coping behaviors; and most importantly, receive regular social interaction. Ultimately, support groups serve as an important forum for teaching and learning, and promoting good citizenship by helping each other.

Generally interventions focus on physical and observable recovery, but perhaps equal consideration should be directed toward *emotional rehabilitation,* which addresses facing the reality of the here and now, where the self-image matches the mirror image. All patients expect to recover because previous experiences with other illnesses have taught them that recovery is the ultimate outcome of other major or minor illnesses. Even knowing someone else who survived a CVA or TBI and did not recover does not prepare an individual for the physical changes that have taken place. Routine familiar and comfortable skills and activities have been altered, and this induces a sense of discomfort, loss of independence, and thus battered self-image. Patients struggle to regain a balanced perspective of new reality where lifelong plans and goals have changed and they are forced to seek alternatives; their identity is now reduced to relationships: wife, mother, daughter, sister, or friend and the activities and profession that defined their independence is altered for the rest of their life. Emotional rehabilitation may take months or years to achieve, and it results from compensating for the losses, building a new self-image and self-esteem and eventual peace.

SUMMARY

Typically, a rehabilitation team may consist of any of the following professionals: speech-language pathologist, physical therapist, occupational therapist, vocational counselor, recreation therapist, neuropsychologist, education specialist and physician. Collectively, their goal is to effect an improvement in the impaired functions through their respective clinical expertise. Apparently "quality of life" is a common issue for all individuals: young and old, brain-damaged and nondamaged. Some degree of curiosity, sense of adventure, desire to learn and meet new people persist among all groups of individuals. The information age and electronic media has enhanced our sense of active participation in the health of our mind and body. It is therefore appropriate to seek answers to pharmacological issues pertaining to the necessity, consequence and dosage of prescribed medications, and also explore alternative forms of interventions.

Advances in tissue culture and cell implantation, and development of synthetic proteins that mimic natural neurochemicals portray an optimistic future for brain recovery. Close to home, individuals with communication disorders should be fostered to seek assistance from diverse health care professionals and family members (or caregivers) to help them overcome their functional deficits. These individuals tend to select respective caregivers for select needs and information and therefore, all professionals play an important role in the recovery process: the common linkage is communication since the majority of our typical day is spent in listening, talking, reading, and writing.

BIBLIOGRAPHY

Adamovich, B. (1998). Functional outcome assessment of adults with traumatic brain injury. *Seminars in Speech and Language, 19,* 281–288.

Alarie-Bibeau, L., and Andrianopoulos, M. (2003, November). *Role of the VL thalamic nucleus in cognitive-linguistic functions.* Paper presented at the meeting of the American Speech-Language-Hearing Association, Chicago, IL.

Albert, M., Goodglass, H., Helm, N., Rubens, A., and Alexander, M. (1981). *Clinical aspects of dysphasia.* New York: Springer-Verlag Wien.

Allen, J., Bruss, J., and Damasio, H. (2004). The structure of the human brain. *American Scientist, 92,* 246–253.

American Speech-Language-Hearing Association. (1987). The role of speech-language pathologists in the habilitation and rehabilitation of cognitively impaired individuals: A report of Committee of Language, subcommittee on cognition and language. *Asha, 29,* 53–55.

Basso, A., Capitani, E., and Vignolo, L. (1979). Influence of rehabilitation on language skills in aphasic patients. *Archives of Neurology, 36,* 190–196.

Bayles, K. and Tomoeda, C. (1991). *Arizona Battery for Communication Disorders of Dementia.* Tucson, AZ: Canyanlands Publishing.

Bellugi, U., Poizner, H. and Klima, E. (1983). Brain organization for language: Clues from sign aphasia. *Human Neurobiology, 2,* 155–170.

Benson, F. and Ardilla, A. (1996). *Aphasia: A clinical perspective.* New York: Oxford University Press.

Benton, A. (1992). *The Revised Visual Retention Test* (5th edition). San Antonio, TX: Psychological Corporation.

Benton, A. (1998). Pitres and amnesic aphasia. *Aphasiology, 2,* 209–214.

Bhatnager, S. (2002). *Neurosciences for the communication disorders* (2nd edition). Baltimore, MD: Williams and Wilkins.

Bower, J. and Parsons, L. (2003). Rethinking the "lesser brain." *Scientific American, 289* (8), 51–57.

Brindley, P., Copeland, M., Demain, C., and Martyn, P. (1989). A comparison of the speech of ten chronic Broca's aphasics following intensive and nonintensive periods of therapy. *Aphasiology, 3,* 695–708.

Cahill, L. (2005). His brain, her brain. *Scientific American, 29* (5), 40–47.

Chapey, R. (Editor). (2001). *Language intervention strategies in aphasia and related neurogenic communication disorders* (3rd edition). Philadelphia, PA: Lippincott, Williams and Wilkins.

Cherepski, M. and Drummond, S. (1987). Linguistic description in nonfluent aphasia: Utilization of pictograms. *Brain and Language, 30,* 285–304.

Coelho, C., DeRuyter, F., and Stein, M. (1996). Treatment efficacy: Cognitive-communicative disorders resulting from traumatic brain injury. *Journal of Speech and Hearing Research 39,* S5–S17.

Code, C. and Müller, D. (Editors). (1983). *Aphasia therapy.* London, UK: Edward Arnold Ltd.

Dabul, B. (2000). *The Apraxia Battery for Adults* (2nd edition). Austin, TX: Pro-Ed.

Damasio, A. (2002). Remembering when. *Scientific American, 288* (9), 66–73.

Davis, A. (2000). *Aphasiology: Disorders and clinical practice.* Boston, MA: Allyn and Bacon.

Dronker, N. (1997). A new brain region for coordinating speech articulation. *Nature, 384,* 159–161.

Drummond, S. (1986). Characterization of irrelevant speech: A case study. *Journal of Communication Disorders, 19,* 175–183.

Drummond, S. and Boss, M. (2004). Functional communication screening in individuals with traumatic brain injury. *Brain Injury, 18,* 41–56.

Drummond, S. and Simmons, T. (1995). Linguistic performance of female aphasic adults during group interaction. *Journal of Neurolinguistics, 9,* 47–54.

Fields, D. (2004). The other half of the brain. *Scientific American, 290* (4), 56–61.

Folstein, M., Folstein, S., and McHugh, P. (1975). "Mini mental state." *Journal of Psychiatric Research, 12,* 189–198.

Frattali, C., Thompson, C., Holland, A., Wohl, C. and Ferketic, M. (1995). *Functional Assessment of Communication Skills for Adults.* Rockville, MD: American Speech-Language-Hearing Association.

Friederici, A., Hickok, G. and Swinney, D. (Guest Editors). (2001). Brain imaging and language processing (Special Issue). *Journal of Psycholinguistic Research, 30* (3).

Goldstein, K. (1942). *After effects of brain-injuries in war: Their evaluation and treatment.* New York: Grune and Stratton.

Goodglass, H., Kaplan, E. and Barresi, B. (2000). *Boston Diagnostic Aphasia Examination* (3rd edition). Hagerstown, MD: Lippincott, Williams and Wilkins.

Grant, D. and Berg, E. (1993). *Wisconsin Card Sorting Test.* Tampa, FL: Psychological Assessment Resources.

Hacke, W., Henerici, M., Gelmers, H., and Kramer, G. (1991). *Cerebral Ischemia.* New York: Springer-Verlag.

Hagen, C., and Malkmus, D. (1979, November). *Intervention strategies for language disorders secondary to head trauma.* A short course presented at the annual meeting of the American Speech-Language-Hearing Association, Atlanta, GA.

Hagen, C., Malkmus, D. and Durham, P. (1979). *Rehabilitation of the head injured adult: Comprehensive physical management.* Downey, CA: Professional Staff Association of Ranchos Los Amigos Hospital.

Haines, D. (2004). *Neuroanatomy: An atlas of structures, sections and systems* (6th edition). Philadelphia, PA: Lippincott, Williams and Wilkins.

Helm-Estabrooks, N. and Albert, M. (2004). *Manual of aphasia therapy* (2nd edition). Austin, TX: Pro-Ed.

Helm-Estabrooks, N., Ramsberger, G., Nicholas, M. and Morgan, A. (1989). *Boston Assessment of Severe Aphasia.* Austin, TX: Pro-Ed.

Holland, A. (1980). *Communicative abilities in daily living.* Baltimore, MD: University Park Press.

Holloman, A., and Drummond, S. (1991). Perceptual and acoustic analyses of phonemic paraphaisas in nonfluent and fluent dysphasia. *Journal of Communication Disorders, 24,* 301–312.

Hooper, H. (1983). *The Hooper Visual Organization Test.* Los Angeles, CA: Western Psychological Services.

Howard, D. and Hatfield, F. (1987). *Aphasia therapy: Historical and contemporary issues.* London,

UK: Lawrence Erlbaum Associates, Publishers.

Hydrocephalis Association (2002). *About normal pressure hydrocephalus—A book for adults and their families.* California: San Francisco.

Jakobson, R. and Halle, M. (1956). *Fundamentals of language.* The Hague: Mouton and Company.

Javitt, D. and Coyle, J. (2004). Decoding schizophrenia. *Scientific American, 290* (8), 48–55.

Kaplan, E., Goodglass, H., and Weintraub, S. (2001). *The Boston Naming Test* (2nd edition). Philadelphia, PA: Lippincott, Williams and Wilkins.

Keenan, J., and Brassell, E. (1975). *Aphasia Language Performance Scale.* Murfreesboro, TN: Pinnacle Press.

Kertesz, A. (1982). *Western Aphasia Battery.* San Antonio, TX: Psychological Corporation.

Kertesz, A. (1996, November 13). *Primary progressive aphasia.* A televised presentation (Teleround 33) sponsored by the National Center for Neurogenic Communication Disorders, Tucson: University of Arizona.

Kiernan, J. (2005). *The human nervous system: An anatomical viewpoint* (8th edition). Philadelphia: Lippincott Williams and Wilkins.

Landauer, T. and Bjork, R. (1978). Optimal rehearsal patterns and name learning. In M. Gruneberg, P. Morris, and R. Sykes (Editors), *Practical aspects of memory* (pp. 625–632), London: Academic Press.

LaPointe L. and Horner, J. (1979). *Reading comprehension battery for aphasia.* Austin, TX: Pro-Ed.

Levin, H., O'Donnell, V., and Grossman, R. (1979). The Galveston orientation and amnesia test: A practical scale to assess cognition after head injury. *Journal of Nervous and Mental Disorders, 167,* 675–684.

Libby, P. (2002). Atherosclerosis: The new view. *Scientific American, 288* (5), 46–55.

Luria, A. (1980). *Higher cortical functions in man* (2nd edition). New York: Basic Books.

McElduff, K, and Drummond, S. (1991). Communicative functions of automatic speech in nonfluent aphasia. *Aphasiology, 15,* 265–278.

McNeil, M., and Presscott, T. (1978). *Revised Token Test.* Baltimore, MD: University Park Press.

Meltzer, C., Kondziolka, D., Villemagne, V., Wechsler, L., Goldstein, S., Thulborn, K., Gebel, J., Elder, E., DeCesare, S., and Jacobs, A. (2001). Serial [18F] Fluorodeoxyglucose positron emission tomography after human neuronal implantation for stroke. *Neurosurgery, 49,* 586–592.

Merci Retrieval System (2005, March 21). *Concentric Medical website,* http://concentric-med ical.com/products_retrieval.html.

Minkowski, M. (1963). *Problems of dynamic neurology.* Jerusalem, Israel: University Hospital and the Hebrew University Hadassah Medical Science.

Nolte, J. and Angevine, Jr., J. (2000). *The human brain in photographs and diagrams* (2nd edition). St. Louis: Mosby.

Norris, M. and Drummond, S. (1998). Communicative functions of laughter in adult aphasia. *Journal of Neurolinguistics, 11,* 391–402.

Petri, H. and Mishkin, M. (1994). Behaviorism, cognitivism and the neuropsychology of memory. *American Scientist, 82,* 30–37.

Pimental, P. and Kingsbury, N. (1989). *Mini inventory of right brain injury.* Austin, TX: Pro-Ed.

Poeck, K., Huber, W., and Willmes, K. (1989). Outcome of intensive language treatment in aphasia. *Journal of Speech and Hearing Disorders, 54,* 471–478.

Porch, B. (1981). *Porch Index of Communicative Ability* (3rd edition). Palo Alto, CA: Consulting Psychologists Press.

Ramachandran, V. and Hubbard, E. (2003). Hearing colors, tasting shapes. *Scientific American, 289* (5), 53–59.

Raven, J. (1995). *Raven's Coloured Progressive Matrices.* San Antonio, TX: Psychological Corporation.

Reisberg, B., Ferris, S., DeLeon, M. and Crook, T. (1982). The Global Deterioration Scale for assessment of primary degenerative dementia. *American Journal of Psychiatry, 139,* 1136–1139.

Research Foundation (1990). *Guide for use of the Uniform Data Set for medical rehabilitation.* Buffalo, NY: State University of New York.

Rosenbek, J. (1985). Treating apraxia of speech. In Johns, D. (Editor), *Clinical management of neurogenic communicative disorders* (2nd edition) (pp. 267–312). Boston, MA: Little, Brown and Company.

Ross-Swain, D. (1996). *Ross Information Processing Assessment.* Austin, TX: Pro-Ed.

Sands, E. and Fitch-West, J. (1987). *Bedside evaluation screening test for aphasia.* Aspen Publishers.

Sapolsky, R. (2003). Taming stress. *Scientific American, 289* (5), 89–95.

Sarno, J., Rusk, H., Diller, L., and Sarno, M. (1972). The effect of hyperbaric oxygen on the mental and verbal ability of stroke patients. *Stroke, 3,* 10–15.

Sarno, M., Silverman, M., and Sands, E. (1970). Speech therapy and language recovery in severe aphasia. *Journal of Speech and Hearing Research, 13,* 607–623.

Sarno, M. and Levita, E. (1971), Natural course of recovery in severe aphasia. *Archives of Physical Medicine and Rehabilitation, 52,* 175–178.

Sarno, M. and Levita, E. (1981). Some observations on the nature of recovery in global aphasia after stroke. *Brain and Language, 13,* 1–12.

Schuell, H., Jenkins, J. and Jimenez-Pabon, E. (1964). *Aphasia in adults.* New York: Harper and Row.

Selim, J. (2002). The biology of handedness. *Discover, 23* (1), 30–31.

Shewan, C. (1978). *Auditory comprehension test for sentences.* Chicago, IL: Biolinguistics Clinical Institutes.

Shewan, C. and Bandur, D. (1986). *Treatment of aphasia: A language-oriented approach.* San Diego, CA: College-Hill Press.

Shewan, C. and Kertesz, A. (1984). Effects of speech and language treatment on recovery from aphasia. *Brain and Language, 23,* 272–299.

Shreeve, J. (1995). The brain that misplaced its body. *Discover, 16* (5), 82–91.

Skelly, M. (1979). *Amer-Ind gestural code based on universal American Indian hand talk.* New York: Elsevier.

Sklar, M. (1973). *Sklar Aphasia Scale.* Los Angeles, CA: Western Psychological Services.

Snell, R. (2001). *Clinical neuroanatomy for medical students* (5th edition). Philadelphia: Lippincott, Williams and Wilkins.

Teasdale, G., and Jennett, B. (1974). Assessment of coma and impaired consciousness. *Lancet, 2,* 81–84.

Teicher, M. (2002). Scars that won't heal: The neurobiology of child abuse. *Scientific American, 288* (3), 68–75.

Templer, D., Hartlage, L., and Cannon, W. (Editors) (1992). *Preventable brain damage: Brain vulnerability and brain health.* New York: Springer Publishing Company.

Tikofsky, R (1971). Two studies of verbal learning by adult aphasics. *Cortex, 7,* 105–125.

Van Lancker, D. and Sidtis, J. (1992). The identification of affective-prosodic stimuli by left- and right-hemisphere-damaged subjects: All errors are not created equal. *Journal of Speech and Hearing Research. 35,* 963–970.

Wepman, J. (1951). *Recovery from aphasia.* New York: Ronald Press Company.

Wepman, J. (1972). Aphasia therapy: A new look. *Journal of Speech and Hearing Disorders, 37,* 203–214.

Wertz, R., Collins, M., Weiss, D., Kurtzke, J., Friden, T., Brookshire, R., et al. (1981). Veterans Administration cooperative study on aphasia: A comparison of individual and group treatment. *Journal of Speech and Hearing Research, 24,* 580–594.

West, J., Sands, E. and Ross-Swain, D. (1998). *Bedside evaluation screening test.* Austin, TX: Pro-Ed.

Wuethrich, B. (2001). Getting Stupid. *Discover, 22* (3), 58–63.

Wylie, C. (1970). The value of early rehabilitation in stroke. *Geriatrics, 25,* 107–113.

INDEX

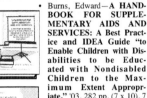

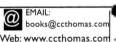
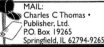